Becoming a mother is a huge life change and sometimes a complete upheaval of all that is familiar. This is a book I highly recommend to mothers and mothers-to-be. It is like an insightful friend who understands deeply what becoming and being a mother really means; the joys and challenges, the journey of discovery through uncharted waters that every mother has before her at each stage of the journey through pregnancy, birth and beyond. It is not a book that gives instructions or makes any assumptions; yet it is very informative, encouraging and above all realistic, with wonderful guidance for making the inner transformation that enables us to grow into motherhood with wisdom, awareness and love. Naomi Chunilal writes from the depth of her personal life journey. Her passion and perception blend in a guide that is truthful and inspiring. Every mother will recognize and find herself in this book.
—**Janet Balaskas**, founder of Active Birth movement, author of *Active Birth*, *The Encyclopedia of Pregnancy and Birth* and *The Waterbirth Book*

Naomi's book is timely and much needed. It is inspiring and encouraging, realistic and open-hearted. She addresses the deep challenges and joys of mothering from a truly profound perspective, and I am sure her book will be of huge benefit to any woman who ever pauses to think about just what it is we are trying to do when we mother our children. Thank you Naomi for your valuable gift to mothers everywhere.
—**Uma Dinsmore-Tuli**, founder of Womb Yoga movement, author of *Mother's Breath*, *Yoni Shakti* and *Yoga for Pregnancy and Birth*

This book is great! A book you will keep referring to for help to inspire a spiritual mindful practice in the day-to-day of motherhood. Labour is really the easiest part of becoming a moth‹ Y, as she traverses the terrain of mothe‹ . A book full of gems and aha momen‹ d practices to keep you connected to y‹ ily.
—**Nadia Narain**, head of Pregnancy Yoga, Triyoga, London

An essential guide every woman will benefit from reading, as she moves on her journey through pregnancy and into motherhood. This book is full of helpful strategies for coping during difficult times with enlightening and inspiring words, so that you can fully embrace and make the most of your pregnancy. It will encourage and empower you to think about your new role as a mother in a unique, more mindful way, and the important part you play in the glorious process of creation as you bring new life into the world.

—**Tara Lee**, leading pregnancy and postnatal teacher, The Life Centre, London, Registered senior teacher with the Yoga Alliance and author of *Pregnancy Health Yoga, Pregnancy Yoga* DVD, *Elements of Yoga, Elements of Yoga: Earth Foundations* DVDs

# the

# mindful

A Practical and Spiritual Guide to Enjoying
Pregnancy, Birth and Beyond with Mindfulness

# mother

Naomi Chunilal

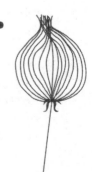

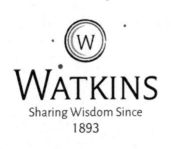

WATKINS

Sharing Wisdom Since
1893

This edition first published in the UK and USA 2015 by
Watkins, an imprint of Watkins Media Limited
19 Cecil Court
London WC2N 4EZ

enquiries@watkinspublishing.co.uk

1 3 5 7 9 10 8 6 4 2

Designed and typeset by Clare Thorpe

Printed and bound in Europe

A CIP record for this book is available from the British Library

ISBN: 978-1-78028-874-1

www.watkinspublishing.com

**Publisher's note:** The information in this book is not intended as a substitute for
professional medical advice and treatment. If you are pregnant or are suffering from any
medical conditions or health problems, it is recommended that you consult a medical
professional before following any of the advice or practice suggested in this book.
Watkins Media Limited, or any other persons who have been involved in working on this
publication, cannot accept responsibility for any injuries or damage incurred as a result of
following the information, exercises or therapeutic techniques contained in this book.

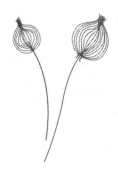

*For my children*
*Sacha and Anouska Rose,*
*With love and blessings.*
*Thank you for choosing us.*

*Close your eyes and you will see clearly.*
*Cease to listen and you will hear truth.*
*Be silent and your heart will sing.*
*Seek no contacts and you will find union.*
*Be still and you will move forward on the tide of the spirit.*
*Be gentle and you will need no strength.*
*Be patient and you will achieve all things.*
*Be humble and you will remain entire.*

**Taoist poem**

Thank you to my dearest friends for their love and honesty in raising an eyebrow or two when necessary, keeping me laughing, trusting and believing, come what may. I would also like to express deep appreciation to everyone who comes to my yoga classes, enriching and teaching me so much by your presence. Thank you for exploring your yoga practice with me.

It goes without saying that I am truly grateful to everyone at Watkins Publishing: in particular Michael Mann for believing in the manuscript, Sandy Draper for making the copy-editing process a pleasure, Clare Thorpe for beautiful design, and Deborah Hercun for expertly guiding *The Mindful Mother* toward publication. Also, everybody else who has helped to affirm the book's message and take it out into the world beyond in some way. In particular, Janet Balaskas, Active Birth Foundation, and Uma Thuli Dinsmore, Womb Yoga, for positive words, kindness and encouragement; and Nadia Nahrain, Triyoga and Tara Lee, The Life Centre, for invaluable feedback and support. Thank you to each and every one of you.

Last of all, my love and thanks to my family who grow alongside me: Jules, my husband, for looking at the stars, the sun rising and walking in the rain; and Sacha and Anouska Rose, our children, for sheer wonder, delight and joy in your presence. For waking us up again and again!

My final acknowledgement is for my parents: my father who found contentment in simple things, trusting in life's benevolence against the odds; coming full circle to my mother, who knows and gives the blessing of boundless love. Thank you for being there.

# CONTENTS

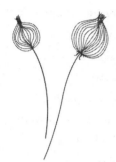

# INTRODUCTION

# AWAKENING MOTHERHOOD WITH MINDFULNESS

*'Our life is shaped by our mind; we become what we think.'*
**Gautama Buddha,** *The Dhammapada*

Motherhood is one of the most immense and life-changing events that can occur in a woman's life. When you give birth, you create a new life, that of your child, and your own as a mother. You start an epic journey of self-discovery and growth that can transform your entire sense of self and identity, not just now, but throughout the rest of your life.

The birth of a child is a profound rite of passage with immense potential to bring infinite joy, delight and enchantment in its wake. Your relationship with your unborn child may be one of the greatest love affairs that you ever have, stretching across decades of your life. It doesn't matter whether you planned this pregnancy, are taken by surprise, or have walked the path of motherhood before. The magical alchemy of maternal love is one of the most wonderful surprises of becoming a mother – a living, breathing gift nourished and renewed by daily contact and nurture between you and your child.

Yet at the same time as falling in love with your child, you are also cast into the role of full-time guardian, with around-the-clock responsibility for meeting their needs and demands both day and night. As you move through pregnancy into this unknown territory of looking after babies and small children, your entire life can feel as though it has been tossed up into the air, leaving you to catch all the different pieces as they fall down. Except that they no longer seem to fit back into the same place as they did before. And you are left, trying to juggle and keep your new life afloat, while feeling consumed by your new maternal role.

As a new mother, you are making massive physical and emotional adjustments to smoothly integrate your baby into your life, while coping with greater levels of tiredness, stress and exhaustion than you have possibly ever felt before. Simple activities such as having a bath, making a phone call, eating supper, sleeping, or chatting with friends are constantly interrupted, seldom reaching a satisfying conclusion. You don't have much time to do anything else apart from look after your baby; whose contentedness often seems to remain outside your immediate control.

As mothers, we instinctively want the best for our children, to give them a happy and stimulating childhood. At the same time, we also hope to find individual fulfilment through the experience of raising a child. Yes, there will be moments of domestic bliss and harmony when these two ideals coincide. Moments when our children smoothly fit into our internal expectations of how we want family life to be. Just not all of the time! So while it goes without saying, that we adore these little people who share our life, it's also true to say that it's not always easy living alongside them. The abrupt reality of giving up autonomy and independence to provide childcare around the clock comes as an immense shock to many of us, often provoking internal conflict and resistance.

So however much you love your baby, they can also seem to destroy your sanity and peace of mind, without doing very much except to open their mouth to remind you they are there. The push and pull of nurture is the fundamental paradox of motherhood. Yet it's easy to forget this, when struggling to keep up with the treadmill of meeting your newborn baby's needs and demands. The relentless nature of looking after a small infant can easily deconstruct your sense of having a normal, functioning adult life. And you may find yourself reacting to anything and everything with frustration, angst, anger and irritability, weepiness and despair. There are times – hours, days, even weeks – when you almost want to turn the clock back to a time before babies were invented!

We so want to make our mothering life calm and upbeat, yet we still manage to collide with countless flash points of stress and tension, often making ourselves, and those around us extremely unhappy in the process. We know that we aren't doing anyone any favours, let alone ourselves, when we forget how to be relaxed and content. Yet it can feel impossible not to feel disappointed, fed up and out of control in the aftermath of this immense life upheaval. There are times when being a mother tests our emotional endurance to breaking point. And we suddenly find our negative emotions are oozing out all over the nursery. And this happens despite our crystal-clear picture of the positive and joyful maternal life that we wish to have.

And so we may sometimes feel that we are barely surviving, and definitely not enjoying ourselves as much as we might like. We hope and expect to have an uplifting experience of motherhood, yet feel unable to notice or appreciate, let alone celebrate the wonder and magic of what is happening in front of our eyes, as we struggle to make our new maternal role comfortably fit into our adult lives.

Yet your individual transition into motherhood holds the seeds of genuine spiritual transformation and growth in its wake. The daily experience of being a mother can become a conscious practice of mindfulness, as we start to explore our living relationships with our children, partners and others, and most of all with ourselves. Who is this inner voice of self, engaging our attention in constant mental dialogue; and how can we find our way to a place of inner stillness and peace? How can we get our mind to work with us, rather than against us? And what is our heart saying to us when we stop and listen?

When we become receptive to exploring our innermost nature, we start to uncover a heart spring of love, wisdom and truth flowing inside us. This is always there, yet can remain buried beneath internal conflict, suffering and tension. When we step onto the path of conscious mothering, our life energy starts to move more easily, and we can see and appreciate who and what we are. With all our imperfections, sorrows and joys. Motherhood and family life becomes a spiritual backdrop against which we can get to know and understand ourselves, and grow, through the simple act of being with our children.

At the same time, our children learn so much about themselves, in the reflection of our life within their own. They witness the world in our relationships with them, and with our partner, friends and family. So it follows that when we feel harmonious, whole and in touch with our higher wisdom and truth, we are more ready and able to guide our children. It is therefore up to you to sow the seeds of your physical, emotional and spiritual awakening into your daily mothering experience.

Mothering can be a daily act of inspiration and grace. We can use daily family life as an emotional catalyst, empowering us to find and cultivate new depths of love and compassion, self-awareness, forgiveness, courage, altruism, self-acceptance, affirmation and resilience.

To become a mother with mindfulness is to celebrate your life. To transform it into a living affirmation, as you accept and embrace whom you truly are, by learning to survive and blossom through the incredible, yet chaotic and often tedious, daily rhythm of life with babies and small children. Having a child now becomes a beautiful and profound rite of passage of awakening consciousness, through the everyday experience of mothering life.

This is about you: your inner journey of spiritual growth and development, as you understand and become the mother you truly want to be to your child.

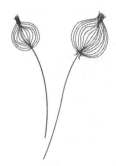

# STEPPING INTO
# PREGNANCY

*'The journey of one thousand miles begins with one step.'*
**Lao Tzu**

P regnancy is a miracle of life and new beginnings. When you discover that you are pregnant, you open an unknown door inside you. Stepping across its threshold, you begin to move into a new chapter of life, as your mind and body starts to grow and change to make space for the unborn baby developing inside your womb. Each day draws you closer to the moment when you will give birth to this child, letting go of your old sense of self and identity to be reborn as a mother.

Yet this passage of nine months is so much more than time spent waiting for your baby to be born. It is the start of your own unique journey into motherhood; a natural breathing space in which to consciously prepare yourself for the profound changes that the birth of a child will bring into your life. Your pregnancy is a wonderful opportunity to slow down, reconnect to yourself and reappraise, appreciate and celebrate your life as you live it.

## So where are you at right now?

The first thing to get your head around is that you actually are pregnant! This may sound obvious, but when you are still staring at the blue line on your home pregnancy testing kit, you may struggle to accept that this really is happening to you. Until your body shows visible signs of another life existing inside your womb, you may wonder whether you read the test instructions back to front, or imagined the whole thing, because surely you can't be pregnant. Except that you are of course!

To become pregnant is immense, groundbreaking news that may feel wonderful and terrifying in equal measures. Since that moment of conception when a certain sperm met the fertile egg inside your uterus, your body is now switched onto pregnancy autopilot that will continue until you give birth. Your body is operating on a massive program of physiological adjustment to support the healthy growth and birth of the foetus developing inside your womb. And your mind and body may react to this new state of affairs in ways you just don't recognize. Your life reduced to trying to cope with alternate waves of intense nausea and cravings on a rollercoaster of changing emotions.

So while you officially know that you are pregnant in theory, you can only guess at the huge impact and upheaval that this fact will have in defining and influencing the rest of your life. You may insist that your offspring will seamlessly morph into your current lifestyle, like a natural offshoot of your existing limbs. Yet you can sense how your unborn child's presence, (even if they are still only of microscopic proportions) is already shifting your entire perspective of what really matters and is important to you.

Your body knows exactly what needs to be done to grow a baby, and is busy getting on with doing this. Yet while your heart may willingly expand into this new realm of babies, your mind may flatly refuse to follow or accept your new status quo as a mother-to-be. So you are pregnant. But how can you help yourself to enjoy and connect to your first steps of the unique rite of passage into motherhood.

## Allowing your mind to catch up

Your pregnancy is a monumental landmark in your life. You will experience moments of sheer joy, peace and bliss during the next nine months as you develop deep bonds of love and empathy for your unborn child. However, you may be surprised, confused and upset to find out you are also feeling a certain amount of internal conflict and resistance about becoming a mother. You expect and want to feel delight, excitement and elation about having a baby. Yet alongside these uplifting emotions are more complex feelings of shock, stress, anger, doubt, fear and anxiety at the imminent prospect of disruption to your life, as you now know it.

You might think you should ignore any misgivings you feel about having a child, now that you are pregnant. So you resolve to only think 'happy' thoughts and hope that your baby won't notice any wayward bubbles of maternal reluctance floating around your placenta. Yet you will never be able to totally convince yourself that your troublesome thoughts and emotions don't exist, however hard you try to be resolutely positive. If they do, they do! And you won't be able to shoo them away with the sheer force of your willpower and effort alone.

You may truly feel 'help!' this really isn't a great time to bring a child into your life due to financial pressures, career development, lifestyle choices, or concern at a rising world population. You may doubt your innate maternal aptitude and would rather not put this to the living test, at least not for another few years or so. You could easily fill a book of doomsday proportions with all the perfectly valid reasons about why you, of all people, really shouldn't become a parent right now.

Of course, we would all like to have flawless maternal instincts, yet we won't conjure these up by simply ignoring our inner conflict about this new combination-to-be of babies, parenthood and ourselves. You are not going to be a dreadful mother just because you are brave enough to acknowledge your mental reluctance. The opposite! You are developing genuine strength, honesty and courage when you learn to face, accept and resolve where your maternal resistance lies.

### ACKNOWLEDGING AMBIGUITY

You are doing you and your baby a disservice, if you ignore or run away from your fears and concerns about becoming a mother. When you shake the dust out of your anxieties and examine them clearly, you can see them for what they are. Stop and pause before you hit the alarm button. And allow your mind some breathing space to get used to your new status quo of being pregnant.

Allow your thoughts to run their course, without giving yourself a hard time about them. Our different thoughts and feelings come and go like clouds drifting across a clear blue sky. Often they dissolve and return again in new shapes and forms. So just because you feel confused and are tied up in knots at this point, it doesn't mean, given time, that you will always be. These shifting thoughts do not equate to who you are and can be. And soon, your mind will move on somewhere else, to another place.

So although you may be genuinely delighted to be having a baby on some levels, you also want other aspects of your life to continue as they are. This is perfectly normal! Most people would have some misgivings, if they got a letter from a stork, informing them that a newborn baby was due to be delivered to their doorstep in nine months. Just because this baby happens to be gestating inside your belly doesn't make it any easier to get your head around the concept.

It will take time to assimilate the reality that you are pregnant, especially if you didn't plan to contact the stork's order line in the near future. And it makes sense to confront and resolve any central dilemmas that you have about new motherhood right now, rather than waiting until you are in the midst of labour!

## Self-acceptance

This is an opportune time for you to be pregnant and become a mother. If only for one simple reason: that it is happening to you right now. Sure you might have tried to stack the odds to make the arrival of babies more or less likely to occur. Yet new life still arises or doesn't for undecipherable reasons. You cannot decide exactly when the sun shines and plants grow. So too, you can't control the flow of universal consciousness. All you can do is trust in life unfolding as it is.

Our individual wishes will never wholly determine what occurs to us, and when this happens – especially when it comes to the birth of babies. As seen in the heartbreaking experiences of many women who struggle to conceive naturally, the cycle of birth and death is something that lies outside our immediate control. So once you decide to continue with your pregnancy and see things through to your due date, accept your unborn child's precious life for what it is: A gift of the universe.

The starting point of your new maternal role is to accept responsibility for a human life, other than your own. Your unborn baby is utterly dependent upon you, and will continue to be so for many years to come. And at some

> **WHAT DOES IT MEAN TO BECOME A MOTHER?**
> What gifts and qualities do you have to share with your child? How do you think
> you need to grow and change to wholeheartedly enjoy this experience? And where do
> you get stuck? Are you judging yourself against an ideal of unattainable success and
> failure? What are your personal responsibilities in bringing a child into the world?
> What kind of world do you want to see them growing up in? And, most importantly,
> how can you make these aspirations happen?

point, you will have to come to terms with this simple truth. This may take
time and practice. So don't worry if you haven't become a saintly mothering
icon of selflessness overnight. This will not be the last time that you fight
aspects of yourself as a mother. Or wonder if you even want a child over the
next 18 years and beyond – however much you also love them!

## Adapting to your body's changes

As the firsthand witness of your pregnancy, you will already be intimately
aware of the internal changes taking place inside your body. You are the
only person in the entire world who can truly appreciate and savour the
signs of new life fluttering in your growing belly. You also have to cope
firsthand with the not-so-enticing physical side-effects of pregnancy;
morning sickness, varicose veins and heartburn hardly being life experiences
to get too excited about!

At the start of the first trimester, your mind and body takes giant internal
leaps forward to become your baby's home for the next nine months. Your
moods may seem to rise and fall on a tidal wave of emotions, as your mind
tries to keep up with the additional physical demands being made upon
your body. Your hormone levels are also rocketing up, which doesn't help
the cause of emotional equilibrium. So don't be surprised if your mind keeps
dragging you off on a deranged loop-the-loop spiral through the entire
spectrum of your emotions.

However, sooner or later, major headlines settle down to become a new normality. You will acclimatize and hopefully radiate out a golden glow of pregnant health and wellbeing. You start to recognize yourself again inside the new outward curve of your profile. And you regain the energy, balance and humour that you may have temporarily misplaced during the first months of pregnancy mayhem. This is great news, especially if you have been searching for your emotional sanity along with the discarded results of your pregnancy home-testing kit in the wastepaper basket for the last few weeks.

Soon you will be well on the way toward your second trimester and the date of your first scan appointment at the hospital. You no longer collapse in shock or hysteria each time somebody mentions your pregnancy. Even though you may secretly wonder if you will ever be truly ready to become a proper grown-up mother. This more settled middle phase tends to continue until you are well into your final trimester, counting down the weeks, instead of months until your due date. Your baby will then start to grow more rapidly in preparation for birth, and your body literally has to rise to the occasion, expanding outward to take the extra weight.

As you reach the home stretch of your last three months, you may experience new sources of discomfort such as acute fatigue, anaemia, heartburn, disturbed sleep patterns, high blood pressure and leg cramps, to mention but a few. Your moods may swing between polar opposites: happiness and anticipation at meeting your child, along with growing unease at the unavoidable process of labour and childbirth looming ahead of you.

Many women worry about how they are going to cope with giving birth to a baby, and start to imagine worst-case scenarios. You may be a lucky carefree woman, and sail peacefully through the final months of your pregnancy like a beautiful curvaceous boat steaming toward harbor. However, if your mind is wobbling, remember that your body knows how to do this, without needing an instruction manual. So all you can do is support, reassure and strengthen both your mind and body to enjoy and engage with your experience of it, as best as you can.

## Moving forward in your pregnancy

As your pregnancy progresses, you will travel far beyond the old edges of your previous comfort zone. You are moving into an unfamiliar landscape, which can feel a long way from the place where you once were. And this gives you a choice. You can sit and wait complacently for things to return to your old definition of normal, which is never going to happen. Alternatively, you can take your first steps on a parallel inner journey of conscious growth, as you get to know the woman you are now, and the mother you will become.

It is so important to enjoy being pregnant as you live through this reality. And nobody else can do this apart from you! When you wake up to the daily miracle of your life, you flourish and blossom in the truth of 'what is', as your unborn child grows inside you. It is your birthright, along with that of your unborn child's. Your individual experience of growing, birthing and nurturing a baby may well turn out to be wildly different from how you imagined it would be, yet you can always seek out and create inner beauty, vitality and joy from whatever passes through it.

### FINDING OUT HOW YOU ARE

You may feel overwhelmed by your growing list of difficult pregnancy conditions such as heartburn, varicose veins, nausea and backache. It's easy to define how we are in relation to physical discomfort. Yet as long as we focus on what's wrong, our mind makes a habit out of suffering, often reducing our life experiences into one long bout of 'ouches.' When we define ourselves as only half-alive – merely OK, surviving, under-the-weather, so-so – we hold ourselves back to exist at this mediocre setting. So, the next time someone asks, 'how are you?' stop and contemplate how you really 'are,' in relation to your life on the planet. You may find that you are actually so much more and doing so much better than just alright! Smile, laugh, step away, look upward at the sky, jump up and down, do anything to let your energy flow again.

### SURRENDERING TO CHANGE

How can you truly say you are ready to guide a child into adulthood if you don't look inside yourself and try to understand more about your own humanity? Is there time to wait to do this? How can you be so sure that you know yourself, when you are already saying and being something quite different from how you were this morning?

As human beings, we exist in a constant state of internal flux known in yogic texts as *Parinamavada*. Our state of mind and body are subtly changing from moment to moment. We know that nothing in life lasts forever, yet we still try to barricade our minds against our sense of insecurity and impermanence. We are afraid that if we are not fixed, solid and constant, living inside a concrete definition of reality, then we are little more than a fading dream of nothingness. Yet, until you actually become a mother with a baby in your arms, how can you know how things are going to happen, let alone how you will process this. So you might as well accept and embrace this glorious uncertainty of not knowing, as you redefine the old cornerstones of your past existence. There is nothing to know, except that you don't know – yet.

## Finding your Breath

Your breath is the vehicle of universal life force or *Prana*, making the bare flesh and bones of your body dance with conscious life. With each breath, your life energy flows, your stream of consciousness shifts, and your thoughts and emotions change, moving from one impulse to another. As long as you breathe, you are alive. So the quality of your breath is the living barometer of your life force, and has the direct capacity to express and influence your health and wellbeing. This is the healing power of breath.

Now that you are pregnant, your baby is held within the soothing and energetic rhythm of your breath tone. When you breathe deeply, you are bathing yourself and your baby in a sea of fresh oxygen and nourishment. Your breath enables your internal organs to metabolize more effectively, removing the waste products of respiration and metabolic activity from your body. When you inhale, your ribcage rises, creating more space inside your abdomen. When you exhale, you release tension, drawing your awareness back down to earth.

As your pregnancy progresses, listen carefully to your breath tone. You may notice that you sometimes struggle with shallowness and shortness of breath. There is literally less surface area available in your lungs, due to your enlarging uterus pressing up against your diaphragm. Your body will tell you when you need to slow down and relax by how much huffing and puffing you are having to do to breathe easily and freely.

## Crossing the bridge of breath

Our breath can draw the mind and body into a state of equilibrium and balance. When we are aware of our breath, our conscious mind connects to the physical flow of life inside us. Our mind and body quiets down into tranquility, and our breath lengthens and slows down into a relaxed and peaceful rhythm. On the other hand, when we are stressed or agitated, our breath quickens and becomes shallow as the body tenses. Wherever our breath goes, the mind and body will follow. So when we control the quality of our breath tone, we literally influence the state of our mind and body.

If you churn up a pond of clear water, it quickly becomes cloudy and obscure, so you can't easily see down to the bottom. So too, when we agitate the surface layers of the mind with unpleasant thoughts and emotions, we become unable to perceive things as they actually are. We no longer notice anything except the ripples of disturbance spreading out across our life. In becoming more conscious of our breath, our mind naturally becomes still – like a pool of water that reflects what lies deep beneath the surface. We observe the sensation of breath moving in and out of the body, and the mind has little choice but to settle down into a state of clarity, focus and absorption.

We can piece the scattered pieces of our mental energy together like a jigsaw puzzle to reveal infinite lucidity and stillness inside us. Sure, it might take us a few weeks, or even months, to focus clearly on what lies beneath the surface, but sooner or later we will find a more complete picture of what this is. We are coming home to rest in the true nature of mind.

## THE PRACTICE OF BREATH AWARENESS

Observe your natural breath as it moves in and out of your body. Focus on a specific point of your respiration cycle, such as the tip of your nostrils, the rise and fall of your belly, or the movement of your chest. Notice the quality and feel the tone of your breath with each successive inhalation and exhalation. You inhale deeply and your baby absorbs vitality. You exhale, drawing your baby close to your core. You nurture your unborn child with your breath flow, holding them in the gentle rhythm of your life force.

As your breath flows, feel your life energy rising within you – spontaneous, fluid and free, as you breathe without mental effort or exertion. As your breath deepens, your mind quiets and your body relaxes into tranquility. You are no longer mechanically breathing, but consciously connecting your mind to the source of your vitality.

Slowly build up your capacity to concentrate on the sensation of breath moving inside you. Your ego may initially resist being told to slow down and focus on the breath. In fact, your ego will say anything to stop you from paying too much attention to anything it doesn't want you to, so it can merrily wander off into its own random daydreams. Be patient and persistent. Hold your mind steady. If you need to, move and stretch out your body, and bring your concentration back to your breath again and again – even when your ego is trying to distract you and reclaim its control over your attention.

Your mind will soon become receptive to following your breath flow, enabling you to drop more easily into a meditative state of alertness. You will start to welcome this restorative time as it replenishes your mental reserves, and connects to the currents of deeper consciousness running through you.

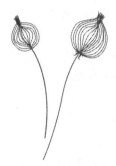

# GETTING TO KNOW
# YOUR PREGNANT SELF

*'Your joy is your sorrow unmasked . . . When you are joyous, look deep into your heart and you shall find it is only that which has given you sorrow that is giving you joy.'*
**Kahlil Gibran**

When you are a child, you instinctively know how to find spontaneous joy and delight through discovering the world around you. Yet as we grow up, our lives become more complex and convoluted. Our natural curiosity slowly suffocates under the weight of adult anxieties, judgment and insecurities. And before we know it, we are limiting ourselves within a straitjacket of attitudes, opinions, beliefs and dogma that dictate and influence our life's purpose.

Except that now, you are pregnant! Your body is working overtime to grow and birth a baby, and your intuitive wisdom knows this is different from your normal expectations of your adult life. Your rhythm of life is changing before your eyes, and confirmed by your softly expanding belly. And this miracle of pregnancy and birth creates a glorious possibility to start afresh and reconnect with all that life can offer you. Your mind and heart are starting to wake up from a deep sleep of complacency to rediscover the world again through the fresh perspective of motherhood.

## Understanding the person we are

We wake up each day, often repeating the same old patterns and cycles of thought and behaviour over and over again. We build up a fragile sense of identity, like a tower of playing cards that could easily topple down with the slightest push. We cling onto the illusion that our personality is something solid that we fix onto us. That this is the way we are, take it or leave it. It helps us to feel more safe and secure, as we navigate our way through an increasingly unpredictable and uncertain world.

Yet we frequently lose our grasp over the control panel in our lives. We try to protect ourselves from the true nature of our human vulnerability by keeping it buried deep inside our hearts. We would prefer to act on autopilot, like a puppet attached to the strings of our habits, rather than admit that we often don't know. In fact we may not have a clue, and aren't always right.

The dense tapestry of our subconscious mind influences what happens to us, often before this even comes to pass. This natural law of cause and effect is what the ancient yogic texts call *Samskara*. We scatter the seeds of intention within our thoughts and emotions, and we harvest the chain of reaction that follows.

In the meantime, we keep on trying to change aspects about ourselves that we dislike; we honestly and truly do. Yet we still keep behaving like an idiot, acting in ways we really don't mean or want to do. We may notice that we are negative or critical, yet struggle to improve certain facets of our relationships with friends or family. There often seems to be precious little that we can do to stop our emotions from taking us off guard, and slamming back into us. Our mental conditioning creates spirals of suffering that we are seemingly unable to fix or change. So while we resolve to make our lives more positive, we keep coming up against ourselves, in spite of our best efforts and intentions. We live as a virtual prisoner trapped inside the hardened shell of our ego; a mechanical human robot set on a repeat program of behaviour in action.

## How the mind weaves thoughts

It may surprise you to notice just how random the mind is. Especially when left to its own devices. Thoughts and emotions flow from one sensory impulse to another in a stream of flowing consciousness, known as the *Vrittis* in yogic texts. We receive a mass of data from the world around us, every

---

**KNOWING WHERE THE MIND IS**

We would all like to think that we know who we are. Yet who is this person who lives inside us, beneath the stream of racing thoughts and emotions? And what actually makes us into the person whom we believe ourselves to be?

Observe what is happening in your mind for a short while. Sit down in a quiet place without distraction, and shut your eyes for a few minutes. Notice how the mind is constantly moving. Do not try to stop or control your stream of consciousness. Just watch how thoughts come and go, as your mind wanders about from one mental stimulus to another. After a few moments, open your eyes.

---

CATCHING HOLD OF THE EGO

Our ego is an integral part of who we are. You will be a happier mother if you can understand and positively shape the impression of how you choose to respond to your children, and can change automatic patterns of behaviour that you don't really want to share with your children. See if you can catch yourself reacting to situations before you even articulate your thoughts and feelings. Dare to stop and change! Think, behave and act differently from how you do out of force of habit. You can catch hold of your ego, and gently harness its power to become a cooperative, willing guide that enables you to live with greater harmony and life purpose.

second that we are alive and exist through our senses. Our mind attempts to organize this jumble of sensory stimuli into some sort of order, largely by filing everything to fit into a self-constructed concept of 'I' and 'me.' That is to say, we relate everything back to ourselves.

Our mind chases after our shifting thoughts and emotions, as if they were something solid and definite, that makes us into us. That would give us a clearly defined outline of personality. If only this was as real and tangible, as we would like it to be. We identify strongly with our individual notion of 'I-am-ness' (known as *Asmita*) to reassure ourselves that we are valid, distinct and do have a reason to exist. So we live inside our ego's limited perspective, fuelled by this hard drive of buried mental patterns and habits. This generates what yogic texts call *Karma* – the wheel of cause and effect. The natural law of *Karma* is neither good nor bad; it all depends on what we choose to manifest in our present, which sets the scene for what will follow us into the future. We become what we think as we take our thoughts out into the world around us.

## Understanding the fight-or-flight response

Most pregnant women agree that their main priority during these nine months is to relax, nourish and nurture themselves, so that they and their baby are cohabiting in a state of optimum health and wellbeing. Yet our stress levels often seem to rise to the contrary during this time, as we turn our lives inside out in preparation for motherhood.

As hunter-gatherers, we successfully overcame the primordial threat of extinction in the natural world around us. We have survived as a species, largely due to our ability to survive dangerous and life-threatening situations through the course of evolution. So when we are placed under stress, our bodies still try to maximize our chances of physical survival, even if this is not strictly necessary.

In modern life, we seldom have reason to hunt for supper. We don't regard ourselves as something to be eaten, and reach for the refrigerator door when we're hungry, and we only tend to see dangerous animals when we visit the zoo. So we rarely have to face genuine life-or-death situations, and have little real need to live on the edge of adrenalin.

Yet the modern brain remains as ready as it ever was, to react to even mildly unpleasant circumstances with a fight-or-flight response. It doesn't matter whether we are facing a genuine threat or not. Our mind shouts 'stress,' and our pituitary gland automatically sends chemical messages to our adrenal glands, releasing stress hormones so we are ready to fight or flee from the potential aggressor. Even if this is only a friendly spider waving its legs at us in the bathtub!

### HOW THE BODY GETS STRESSED

When our mind tells our body to get stressed, we start to react on autopilot to help us safely fight or flee from danger. Our digestive system shuts down temporarily, likewise the immune system. We breathe more shallowly and quickly, enabling our muscles to work overtime to escape from any potential threat to our safety. The pupils dilate and blood gets diverted away to vital organs. Stress doesn't know perspective, so we are automatically led away from a state of balance, healing and equilibrium until the adrenalin stops kicking in.

## Living in tension

We can easily start to believe that we are under constant threat of attack from a hostile world out to get us. And soon, we exist in a habitual state of unresolved tension. We tread an uneasy line between our attack or defense mode, and our adrenal reflex silently feeds off our life force like a parasite. We suppress our body's natural state of homeostasis and weaken our vitality, which can manifest in chronic health problems, such as high blood pressure, low immunity, nervous exhaustion and physical burnout. We can become so preoccupied with the negative symptoms of stress – anxiety, fear, uneasiness, anger, fatigue and restlessness – that we fail to look up or notice that there is often no enemy, except the one we create inside ourselves.

Our mind easily forgets that it doesn't have to operate in stress mode. And there is absolutely no justification for reacting as if the world were about to collapse on our shoulders, when it clearly isn't going to do so. We don't have to cast ourselves as Rumpelstiltskin in our personal life drama, hopping up and down with expert frustration, just because things don't always turn out exactly as we might like. Neither become adept at acting the victim, beating ourselves up for our imperfections.

## Redefining stress

We have a choice: We either get stressed, or not. While we may never remove all of life's difficulties, we can decide how we cope with what is thrown at us. We alone are responsible for ourselves, and for maintaining a positive equilibrium in our lives, regardless of what anyone else says or does to us.

Sure, you may need to make all sorts of important decisions as you contemplate parenthood concerning your career, work, financial security, living arrangements, childcare, friends and extended family's involvement in your life. You may struggle to rearrange the complexities of life around your pregnancy and the prospect of having children, especially when you've previously taken it all for granted as being just so. What matters is that you are open and honest about the difficulties that seem to arise when you explore the sticking points of motherhood. These are genuine concerns, regardless of how trivial, irrational, or just plain mad they seem to be. And now is a time to do something about them. They will then have less power to bother you later on, after giving birth, when you all want to do is nurture your baby in peace, without distractions.

You are being given an amazing opportunity to turn your life inside out, upside down, and mould it into a shape that you want it to be. Your life is truly precious, and will feel the more so, when you open it up and share it with a child. So use the time you have now, to understand what you are choosing to fill it up with. As you voice your worries, fears and anxieties, you dissolve their latent power to hold you in the past, which might otherwise suffocate your power, resolve and motivation to act now. You start to open your heart to face yourself honestly, to see the root causes of stress as they are: something that you don't want or need to include in your mothering plan. Life is already complicated enough, without adding more unnecessary difficulties to carry in it.

Create a mental picture in which you are coping and thriving in a stressful situation. Now take another step forward to believe in and manifest these positive qualities in your life. Only you can give yourself permission to enjoy your pregnancy as it is happens. Alas, you may never remove all of the root causes of tension in your life; in-laws and work may never go away! But you can create an internal toolbox of antidotes to give you enough resilience and coping strategies. This might include a new career path that fits in with your vision of family life, or simply disappearing into the bathroom to shake out waves of irritation at family gatherings.

Smiling and laughing in the face of stress encourages your brain to relax and releases endorphins (the feel-good hormones) throughout your body, and so activates your parasympathetic nervous system. Your mind stops racing, you breathe more easily, boosting your immune system. All of which removes emotional and physical toxicity more effectively from your body. Your baby can now find true refuge living inside your womb.

**LOOSENING LIFE'S STRAIN**

Look at the major components of your life while you are pregnant: partner, children, finances, home, family, friends, work and career. Clarify what is working well for you; and what makes you feel worried and out of sorts. List specific details that you would like to change, breaking these down into simple parts, so you can see exactly what would make your life easier to manage. It's that simple! Now you can identify achievable steps you can take to alleviate stress before it gets a firm grip on you. You may not be able to run away to a desert island to raise a family, but you can discover what can give you greater ease and peace as a mother before you get there.

When we get to know and make friends with the bogeymen who disturb our inner peace, we loosen the tight knot of emotional discord that we hold inside us. We don't get quite so worked up about our personal tales of woe and misfortune unfolding in the soap opera of our lives. We feel more confident and sure-footed about how to leapfrog over obstacles, noticing new possibilities that we didn't even see before. We don't take ourselves quite so seriously, even when we are seriously struggling, and let's face it, stressed! The difference is, we are now choosing our individual response to our life script on our own terms.

## Catching hold of nesting madness

As a mother-to-be, you may be panicking at the prospect of life change. Your immediate response may be to try and reinforce order and control over those aspects of your living circumstances that you can directly influence. Many of us throw ourselves into domestic baby preparations with enthusiastic gusto, like a train gathering steam. We start manically clearing out the clutter in our homes in order to create more newborn baby space. There is, of course, a point to this. No one wants to drown in a sea of baby paraphernalia; especially if you are worrying that you'll need a new extension to store it all.

In shaking the cobwebs out of your surroundings, you make your baby's arrival more tangible and real. Into something that is actually happening to you, rather than an abstract concept. Yet a healthy nesting instinct can rapidly mutate into a hormone-fuelled obsession involving epic proportions of online research and shopping. You start using up vast amounts of time, energy and resources, collecting items from an endless list of 'essential' newborn equipment. Even though you know that your baby won't know or care whether you've got the latest model of infant technology, as long as you are near them. So decide at what point you're going to step off the consumer bandwagon, satisfied with your secondhand buggy and hand-me-down baby clothes, and then stop searching for the missing receipt to a perfect mothering life, thrown away in the packaging around you.

As you sigh with relief at finding a new regime of simplicity, don't get sucked into the second wave of pregnant madness: the great home improvement program to transform your humble abode into a castle. You don't want to loose your newfound time, energy and credit rating in a whirl of domestic ambitions to refit the kitchen, build an extension and redecorate the whole house. All of which is driven by the same hormonal thirst to create a perfect nest around you.

You can put yourself under a lot of pressure to get your surroundings ready for your baby while pregnant. And quickly lose the plot of what really needs to get done. Your pregnancy hormones may try to assert themselves far more forcefully than the quiet wisdom of your common sense asking you to sit down and rest. You don't need to be a slave to unrealistic consumer ideals; namely that a good parent should provide a perfect domestic environment for their offspring. Your home improvement manifesto will never give your newborn infant a more auspicious head start in life, or safeguard their future triumphs and successes.

This child of yours has no choice but to grow up within the emotional ambience you create around you. So, if you suspect you are caught up in a constant flurry of physical activity, give yourself time and space in which to do nothing else, except to be pregnant. Your body is already using up vast amounts of energy, simply by growing a baby. So stop and listen when you are slipping into tiredness, and fill yourself with sufficient rest and nurture.

## Finding resolution

We all struggle with relative schizophrenia at times, dividing ourselves into different personalities with distinct and conflicting priorities. The rational mind often wants to dominate and assume a role of chief foreman, controlling our actions. Then we find that we are continuously busy doing something or other. We tell ourselves that we will stop and relax in just a moment's time, which of course never arrives. In the meantime, we slowly wear ourselves out waiting for life to quiet down a little.

The simple truth is that if you don't slow down, you will start to feel miserable, ill and run down. You will then have to postpone whatever you are doing anyway in order to catch up, recover and redress the balance. However, when you trust and listen to your intuitive health, you develop self-respect and esteem to look after yourself, *and* be a mother, without crumbling away under the pressure.

## Transforming the ordinary

Your pregnancy is a unique time; a deeply profound and individual rite of passage in which to prepare to become a mother. To stop, reflect and

GETTING YOUR LIVING SPACE READY

What are your main priorities in getting your living space ready for your baby, and how much are you doing above and beyond this? Ask yourself honestly, is your latest home-improvement plan strictly necessary, and will it really improve the quality of your life? If you really have to march on with toolbox in hand, then give yourself sufficient rest and nurture when you are tired. And ask for help *before* you need this. Put an equal amount of effort, energy and determination into creating a balanced, healthy lifestyle that reflects how you want to feel right now. Not sometime later at an indeterminate date in the future when you finally put the paint pots away.

appreciate what your life already is. When you give sincere attention to simple acts of 'being,' the heart wakes up, engages and becomes aware. When you repeat the same daily action again with genuine mindfulness, you invest symbolic importance into what you are doing, and give it positive intention. You can continue to enrich mundane routines of life with a deeper resonance, each time that you find emotional satisfaction in doing them. In being present.

You can create a sacred space within the humdrum of everyday existence. There is no obligation to start wearing a white robe; chanting and waving incense sticks to shower blessings upon you and your unborn baby. Unless, of course, you love doing this! But we can always find a deeper appreciation of the vibrant hues, beauty and magic in each day to pass onto our children. In recognizing the divine in our own life, we reaffirm our connection to all other living beings on this planet. We wake up to become present: no longer mechanically marching through the passage of time, but authentically living to the rhythm of our heart's inner truth.

## Leading the mind inward

As long as human life exists, suffering will follow. It should be so simple. You are alive and there is much to enjoy in this. Yet we all get lost trying to carve a definite path of life purpose and happiness out of the impermanence of our lives, especially when people, circumstances and things are constantly changing and evolving around us. It's hard to sustain a peaceful life equation within the sphere of our own human nature. Let alone when we factor in other people's agendas, however much we love and care for them.

It goes without saying that your newborn baby will sometimes challenge your perception of the person you think you are. You are going to come up against your own shortcomings and weaknesses as this tiny human being invades your personal space, innocently rocking your emotional gravity. And you may not always like what you see or find out about yourself. Alas, no woman has yet discovered how to have children without falling off

## SIMPLE ACTS OF RITUAL IN A PREGNANT DAY

As you go about your daily life, slow down and become mindful of what you are doing. Listen to what your heart is telling you, as you go about your life.

The next time you take a bath or shower, wash your body and cleanse your mind of stressful thoughts or feelings, anything that isn't useful that you may be holding onto. As the water flows over you, allow your mind to become fresh and sparkling.

When you are outside, take a few seconds to appreciate the fresh air around you – even if you are only taking out the recycling. As you breathe in, feel your spirits lift and lighten, then breathing out, give gratitude to the earth.

Wherever you are, stop and look closely at something natural, such as a plant, an animal or the landscape. Notice what your eyes are seeing and your ears hearing, without defining what this is, as if you were witnessing life for the first time.

Appreciate and bless the food in front of you when you are eating a meal. Consciously enjoy each and every mouthful, noticing the different tastes, sensations and flavours nourishing you and your baby.

When you next do the housework, wipe away old, congested values, habits and judgments gathering dust within you. As you clean your surroundings, create fresh spaciousness in your thoughts. Don't hurry to finish your chores as quickly as possible, but engage your whole attention in what you are doing at a measured pace.

As you walk, be conscious of planting down each foot on the ground. Notice how your body moves, taking each step with joy and awareness. Allow yourself to stroll at a relaxed pace, rather than rushing to get somewhere as quickly as possible.

a maternal pedestal! You are destined to feel the whole mixed bag of messy human emotions as a new mother. Your own state of mind intensified by the sheer hard work and pressure of swimming in circles around another small person's needs.

## Being present

You are only ever alive in this moment, and so yes, you want to enjoy all of it now when you can. As a mother, this means accepting everything that you are feeling in your new role. Not just the good bits when you and baby appear to be on track, and are set to live happily ever after.

If you ignore the person you really are, you set yourself up to fall down into a waking dream of disappointment. Your emotions will suddenly flip over to reveal raw sensations of vulnerability, suffering and pain. You can't ignore or erase complicated feelings that erupt when things suddenly feel difficult: your baby throws up on the clean bed linen, starts to grizzle when you sit down to eat supper, or unwittingly does something else that touches your nerve endings. To come to terms with the relative opposites of joy and sorrow means accepting everything that you experience. That is *all* of your emotions, not just the positive ones that you like and want to keep. This is the path of inner freedom.

You are already complete, perfect and whole: a microcosm of the entire universe. All you need do is recognize and know the truth of this. After giving birth, you put your old life to rest, and forge out a new reference point of perspective. So, as your life changes around you, it can only help to understand what is going on inside your mind. In creating a meditative path, you start to shift and loosen some of the mental clutter and debris clogging up your perception. You can now see and follow your inner light, illuminating your higher self and true nature far more easily. To arrive in the present of being and be true to whom you are.

## Finding your own meditative path

The mind can become a sanctuary, regardless of what is 'done' to us, on the outside. When we meditate regularly with sincerity and effort, we discover a rich inner harvest of truth, wisdom and insight already growing inside us. So how can we live mindfully, instead of being tossed about by an unruly, uncontainable mind that often refuses to do what we want it to?

Set aside a realistic amount of time to meditate in, anything between 5 and 30 minutes each day to start with. Slowly increase this time, as and when you can. You may find it helpful to sit at a regular time, so your meditation practice gets done, rather than hoping you will find a few minutes time later on in the day. You could set the alarm clock a few minutes earlier in the morning, or meditate after putting children to bed, or before you go to sleep.

There will be days, sometimes weeks, when you don't feel like meditating and can find many more important, urgent things to do. Yes, of course you always need to put out the flames first if your house is on fire. Yet the ego will also delight in conjuring up all sorts of distractions and excuses, often perfectly valid, to try and stop your meditation practice from taking up the centre-stage of attention.

Set yourself a steady pace, meditating patiently and diligently through obstacles. Your mind will start to recognize and welcome this inner space of peace. You will soon become able to drop more readily into a meditative state. Your practice becomes like an anchor that holds the rest of your life afloat and steady.

It doesn't matter if you don't have a dedicated meditation space in your home, complete with candles, soft lights and minimal distraction. As most mothers know, it is often impossible to find personal space of any description, which isn't hijacked by the demands of your offspring, day or night. So, do not let a humble meditation abode that includes your children at its centre, hinder you from turning your mind inward.

You can be mindful every second that you are alive: when you walk to the bus stop, get on the bus, sit down on the bus, and get off the bus again. On the other hand, you might be sitting in paradise with incense burning and statues of the Buddha gazing down at you, and still your mind keeps wandering. You alone can lead your mind into a meditative state of alertness, focus and clarity as you learn to sustain your inner focus on a specific object of contemplation.

It may seem impossible to do this when your partner, baby and children are all clamouring for your attention. Yet this is when you most need to gather up your mental reserves to find meditative stillness and peace. When we relax and let go of our expectations of how we want our lives to be, we can see and appreciate how they actually are. And wake up to cherish the miracle that is already happening.

## CREATING MEDITATION SPACE

Sit upright in a comfortable position. Support your body with pillows or cushions, and gently move whenever you need to. Allow your spine to lift as if someone were gently pulling you up by a cord running through the centre of your body. Shut your eyes, and then softly breathe in and out of your nostrils. Observe your natural flow of breath: a profound meditation practice in its own right.

As your mind slows down, notice your thoughts and feelings skimming over the surface of your awareness. And then let these go and move on. As clouds drift past over a clear blue sky, observe how your thoughts, feelings and sensations come and go, changing by themselves against a spacious backdrop of stillness. Allow yourself to let go of distraction, willpower and effort that try to make this into something else, other than what it is.

## Looking at mental shadows

When we create division between the world outside and inside us, we start to manifest anger, jealously, fear, doubt, insecurity and irritation. We find that we are trapped in negative thoughts, and become disappointed because things don't seem to match up to our hopes and dreams. Our mind may tend to only notice and focus on just one small part of our entire life picture – which may be a negative slant of the situation. So while the letter 'h' can mean 'happiness,' or something positive in a different context, we only manage to notice the 'horrible' aspects around us, according to the angle of our perception. So we remain stuck inside a self-perpetuating judgment that obscures our vision of anything else that lies beyond.

You don't know how you are going to find being a mother until you get there. But you can decide to let go of old negative habits now, for which you will have little positive use. Give yourself a fighting chance to be ready to accept happiness when you meet it. You don't need to find a wordy explanation about why you are doing this. Just step into fresh space, do things differently, and your mind will follow.

When you shine light on your shadows, there is nowhere for them to hide. So the next time that you get stuck in a bog of unhappy, angry, or gloomy thoughts, pick up your inner gaze and literally turn it onto something else. Lift up your thoughts and put them in a different place from where you were back then, to create a new stream of consciousness.

You choose your inner dialogue in every moment that you're awake and conscious. So decide to only dance to the tune of your positive thoughts. You can change your moods in an instant through simple acts that affirm what life is worth to you. Find joy in small things: a small gesture of kindness to a stranger, giving compassion to a friend, smiling at the absurd, noticing glimpses of contentment. The sky is your limit as you find new ways of appreciating the intrinsic divinity and goodness in what already is, inside and around you.

### SHARING LIGHT INSIDE

Lie down or sit comfortably, supporting yourself with pillows and cushions. Become aware of your body resting, your breath moving inside you. Do not try to change or control your breath tone; just let it be as it is.

Scan your body from the crown of your head down over your skull, through your arms, hands, upper body, pelvis, legs and feet. Use your breath to fill yourself up where you feel stagnant or empty. Feel the warmth of your breath dissolving tiredness and tension, smoothing out the edges.

Visualize an orb of golden white light above the crown of your head. Entering your body through the crown, it pours down into you, a stream of light radiating through your body. This pure healing light touches your heart, dissolving any congested energy you are holding within you. You are bathing your internal organs in a sea of golden, white luminosity. As a candle lights up a dark room, your mind and body glow in the warmth of this healing vibration, resonating in every cell and particle of your entire body.

This source of healing energy strengthens with the vibration of your breath flow. As you breathe in, your life force rises up through your body to merge with the stream of light shining above you. As you breathe out, this healing light pours down through your body's axis into the earth. Rest deeply. Before you move on, connect to the source of healing energy in your heart space, knowing that you can always find and use this whenever you need to.

Gently bring your palms together to rest on the heart and give out love and blessings to the universe.

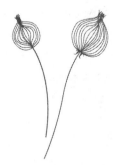

# CONNECTING TO
# YOUR UNBORN BABY

*'Sitting quietly, doing nothing, spring comes,*
*and the grass grows by itself.'*
**Zenrin-Kushu**

Your pregnant body exists in a beautiful relationship with your unborn child. As you surrender to the simple truth of being pregnant, you will feel profound bonds developing between you and your child. Your internal resistance starts to dissolve when your heart opens up to the vulnerable human life growing inside you. This is not to say that you no longer have any concerns or misgivings about becoming a mother. But at base level you are connected to the source of love linking you together.

So when you come to give birth, you will be able to tune into your baby's presence, giving them the reassurance, comfort and strength that they need. You can guide each other through labour, without ever feeling separation – even as your baby is delivered from the safety of your body into your arms, arriving in the world outside.

## Sharing energy

All human relationships are based on an exchange of energy. In giving birth, your body gives life to another human being. At the same time, you receive the gift of this new life in your own. As you breathe deeply, become conscious of your child's presence growing silently inside your womb. Talk and chat to your unborn baby, sing, communicate and get to know them. Your unborn child will become aware of who you really are: soft, vulnerable and exposed with your defences down. Open yourself up to become a loving, accepting presence around them, as you dissolve the boundaries of division between you both.

## Enjoying your growing roundness

A seed obtains its life force from three basic elements in its surroundings: light, nourishment and roots within the earth. When you receive these ingredients in daily abundance, your mind and body flourish and grow. You allow your spirit to dance in life's blessings as you align yourself to a higher truth and purpose. You consciously decide to seek out, appreciate and enjoy life, or else choose to turn away from the source of light into shadow.

## CHANNELING LIFE ENERGY TO YOUR CHILD

Sit or lie down in a comfortable position in a quiet, warm and calm environment, supporting your pregnant body as necessary with pillows and cushions. Shut your eyes and become aware of stillness. Observe the rise and fall of your breath, your heartbeat, digestive system and body at rest. Allow yourself to soften and release every single muscle and tissue group within your body, so that you feel a sense of deep relaxation and peace expanding through you.

Start to visualize your unborn baby growing inside your womb. Concentrate on building up a clear picture of their human form. Focus on all the tiny details of their physical body: their fingernails and toenails, skull and face, limbs, vital organs, the rhythm of their heart beating. Imagine how it is to be living in their world inside the protective sphere of your womb.

Rub your palms together to generate warmth and place your hands gently onto your belly. As you breathe out, imagine that golden-white light is pouring from your palms into every cell and molecule of your entire body. You are bathing your unborn baby in a sea of healing light, holding them safe within your uterus.

Move your hands over your belly, directing your life energy wherever you feel it needs to go. Concentrate your healing intention – compassionate, benevolent and reinvigorating – by focusing on your breath flow energizing your hands. Now place your hands onto your belly again and feel your baby's living presence beneath them. Consciously feel your love growing, expanding toward your baby, and offer this to them.

You can always revitalize your relationship with the changing vehicle of your pregnant body that gives you physical form. This is a great time to either start or reaffirm a conscious habit of mutual care toward you and your baby-in-residence. So you are bathing in pure vital energy at the inception of your shared lives together. This is a gift of love. As you act with a higher intention, you will find there is more love to give and receive inside you.

Each day, you can decide to eat healthy, fresh and nourishing food prepared with attention and care, allowing your body to digest and absorb its nutritional goodness. You might want to make other lifestyle changes: improve your diet, exercise sensibly, and make sure that you rest, relax and sleep well each day. There is nothing in this that you haven't already heard countless times before. Yet when was the last time that you really listened, and then followed the silent cues of your mind, body, or heart? Without ignoring your instinctive wisdom, getting distracted, or doing exactly the opposite.

### LIVING WITH WHOLENESS

Consider whether your life is full of the values you need in order to sustain a calm, peaceful and happy existence. The words you use, the sensory input you choose, the food you take into your body. What do they all add up to? Reduce anything that could be destructive in your life, if possible. Avoid thoughts, words and surroundings that generate a poisonous, harmful and violent ambience, counterproductive to joy and contentment.

*Sauca*, or cleanliness, is the practice of cultivating purity in words and actions. Something that starts in little things that you can actively change. Speaking gently without using words that hurt you or others, eating fresh, healthy food, filling your mind and body with nourishment that uplift your spirits. Give yourself stimulation that enhances your wellbeing; that can do you good, rather than disturb or harm you. Everything has a cause and effect. Start with having a positive influence on your own life, rather than expecting this to happen without your conscious involvement. So then, there is less to disturb the mind's tranquility. You can see what is in you already more clearly, without mental or physical disturbance.

You have nine months to clean up your physical act. Throwing out any old habits of overindulgence, self-negligence and hedonism. You can change, helped by your pregnant body's natural antipathy to a lifestyle of rock-and-roll excess. The option of a healthy and balanced way of life cannot be a half-hearted choice at this point. This needs to become your new daily mantra, empowering you to create positive outcomes in your mothering experiences with your child.

## Owning your pregnancy

The primary focus of modern medical prenatal care is to keep you and your baby safe and healthy before, during and after birth. This is everyone's main objective – most of all your own as a mother. Labour can be unpredictable. And until recently, complications during childbirth could potentially endanger the life of both mother and unborn child. Nowadays, we are immensely blessed to live in a society that has the medical expertise and resources to be able to identify and reduce many of the risk factors previously associated with pregnancy, childbirth and early infancy.

Modern pregnancy healthcare is usually a straightforward process, ensuring you and your baby's healthy growth and development. Your prenatal care normally involves regular physical examinations to assess different aspects of your unborn baby's existence: monitoring the size of fingernails, gender type, circumference of skull, fetal positioning and approximate due date. You will leave your appointments with a lot of reassuring data that helps you to sleep more easily at night, knowing that your baby is healthy, safe and well. Yet you may also feel invisible at prenatal clinic, as a real-life person. Your personal experience is swallowed up in a generic clinical drive that defines and treats your pregnancy as an impersonal medical condition.

Individual medical personnel may personally be kind, well meaning and respectful of the leading role you play as mother-to-be in your pregnancy show. Yet doctors and midwives also have to operate within a tight professional remit and budget constraints. They are professionally bound to focus predominantly on your physiological role as the human baby carrier of the foetus growing in your womb.

You are a strong and powerful individual who can enjoy an awesome, enriching and ecstatic experience of pregnancy, labour and childbirth. Yet you will only make this happen when you trust, want and believe that it can be like this. If you are enjoying a straightforward and uncomplicated pregnancy, then there is no reason why you should not have a say in how you want to do pregnancy and give birth. Your baby needs to be kept safe, and so do you. Beyond this, you don't have to accept whatever medical intervention is on offer on your due date just because it is standard hospital procedure. Unless, of course, this is what you want.

So if you are adamant that you do not want pregnancy and labour to be 'done' to you, then you need to be healthy, strong and emotionally grounded, so that you can make and follow through your decisions and choices. You will then be able and ready to engage in your own pregnancy and labour with all of the mental focus, determination and physical resilience that you have to give it. If you do need to be given extra medical help, then you know that you are accepting this for the right reasons. Namely to proactively safeguard you and your baby's health and wellbeing.

We live in an achievement-orientated world that tends to measure success in absolute and concrete goal-driven terms. And so, the doctor's clinic obviously has to concentrate on fulfilling certain medical procedures driving your prenatal care. Thank goodness that this is so! Yet this needn't be the only litmus test that defines your pregnancy. If you only measure pregnancy and labour in relation to your performance on linear health indices, then you may end up missing much of the intuitive wonder and magic of your baby's gestation, and your own unique role in this.

## Standing tall on the earth

It is your birthright to stand upright – securely planted on the earth's surface – so that you can courageously face whatever life throws at you. Think about the footprint that you are creating on the planet. When you stand and walk tall, you feel confident, better about yourself, and know where you are going. You feel alive and know it! There is every reason to celebrate that you are a unique and wonderful person with amazing gifts and qualities to share with your fellow human beings. So do not slouch and try to hide inside yourself. You have nothing to gain by shrinking or becoming invisible as if you were ashamed to be alive. You have just the one mind and body, and the chance of a single lifespan to fill and use it!

You do not want to wake up after you become a mother and find that you are vulnerable and lost, and you no longer know who you are. By deepening your roots now with the earth, you are cultivating new reserves of inner strength that will hold you secure and steady, even as your external façade of life changes around you.

## Preparing your body for childbirth

After your first trimester of pregnancy, you may decide to attend an antenatal yoga or birth-preparation class. Do you need to do this? Well, would you run a marathon without any sort of prior training? Of course not! Active labour is a similarly intense feat of physical endurance, often lasting for hours, which also requires you to tap into an inner reservoir of courage, strength and resilience. After which, you need to recuperate and recover as quickly as possible to get on with looking after your baby. Do not underestimate the challenge that lies ahead of you!

A dedicated pregnancy yoga and birth preparation class will help to increase your physical and emotional capacity, to manage your own pregnancy and labour process. Through gentle physical, mental and breathing exercises, you will learn how to strengthen specific muscle groups associated with childbirth while connecting with your unborn child. You

## LIVING WITH MOUNTAIN-LIKE PRESENCE

Stand upright with your feet placed hip-width apart. Flex and lift up your toes, replanting them back down one by one, from the outer edges in toward the big toe. The soles of your feet spread out, anchoring your pregnant body to the earth's surface. Strengthen your legs by drawing energy up through the arches of your feet, calves, kneecaps and thigh muscles – to the base of your pelvis. Allow your spine to naturally lengthen and create more abdominal space. Draw your chin in to relax the muscles along the sides and back of your neck. As you release your shoulder blades downward, your chest opens and your arms and hands hang lightly down on either side.

Your breath fills every molecule, tissue and organ of your body. Stabilize your centre of gravity inside your pelvis, creating strong roots through your legs and feet into the earth. At the same time, gently reach up through your spine to the crown of your head. As you breathe in and out, cultivate secure and deep foundations with the ground under your feet, even while your mind opens and soars in the universe.

may soon find that yoga becomes a powerful life support that carries you over the mountains of pregnancy, labour and childbirth and through the rest of your mothering life.

## Finding your place in the universe

Your relationship with the universe gives you life: providing you with sunshine, food and water, shelter, and fresh air to breathe. Your life force arises from this great river of consciousness. You can never exist only as the solitary letters of your name written on a birth certificate. Like a drop of water that merges into a stream to join the ocean, you are an inseparable part of the whole living organism of existence.

The living thread of your breath supports you, to take in and release what you need, in order to sustain your individual life on the planet. As you breathe in, you create a new beginning. You cannot hold onto your last breath. It is already gone; it is no longer there. There is a chance to start again and again; to resolve, let go, and be reborn in each breath you take. You breathe out and loosen the grip of old habits, judgments and ideas holding you back from new possibilities. There is nothing to fear and everything to discover about the microcosm of the universe already existing inside you.

## Living with the seasons

The seasons of nature slowly pass as days, weeks, months come and go. Your unborn child will mature and grow until they are ready to be born. Listen to the natural cycle of your life force, and respect this as it ebbs and flows. There is a perfect time for your body to rest, sleep and wake, rather than following a diary of engagements. Your mind chatters and clamours to keep on track with your schedule, yet your body wants something else. Your life is sustained by the quiet internal rhythm of nature unfolding inside and around you. So listen gracefully to your intuition and become receptive and accepting of whatever comes to pass.

## The healing power of touch

Massage is a relaxing tonic for your body – soothing the nervous system and calming the senses. As your baby's weight increases, your body is constantly adapting to this growing pressure on its resources. So a professional or home massage is a wonderful support mechanism, which is able to uplift your mind and body when it is working overtime. This will help to alleviate some of the more difficult side-effects of pregnancy: releasing tired muscles, stimulating circulation and lymph flow back to the heart, and promoting homeostasis. When you are cocooned inside this sensual space, you can switch off other responsibilities, catching up with where your mind and body are at in relation to becoming a mother.

USING MASSAGE

Self-massage creates a tangible bond between you and your baby inside your uterus. Sit down in a warm comfortable place. Smooth some massage oil, such as wheatgerm or sweet almond oil over your belly. Enjoy the shape of your beautiful, growing roundness, massaging the soft contours of your body wherever you need this. There is no right or wrong way to give a massage, and you will know what feels right for you. As your hands meet the living form of your baby, take time to connect to them as a real person, nurturing yourself and them with sensual care and attention.

## Welcoming your unborn baby

You may want to create a simple ceremony to mark your pregnancy, gathering close friends and family around you to witness your birth into motherhood. The support and blessings of those people whom you love, respect and trust can be an amazing source of strength and inspiration as you grow through this special rite of passage. Creating a community around you of people you love, who will cherish and nurture your child's life.

Think about your underlying intentions behind the structure and flow of this ceremony. You could decorate and cleanse a special space, burning essential oils that have purifying properties, such as juniper, frankincense, or cedar wood. You might want to create a visual focal point, such as lighting a bonfire, or setting out a special table on which people can place symbolic objects of meaning to you both. Reflect on what you share with each of your guests, and ask them if they would like to bring something special to mark the occasion. You could ask participants to choose a poem, song, dance, music, visualization, or meditation that will inspire you through the coming months. You might also prepare and share a meal with your guests. This is your pregnancy, yours alone, and nobody else's. So only invite people who will support you through this.

## Dipping into pregnancy celebrations around the world

There is a strong lineage of women around the world who believe in honouring their rite of passage into motherhood through the art of ceremony. There are many beautiful traditions, based upon universal principles: making offerings to mother earth, asking for the universe's protection, expressing blessings and gratitude, and creating a safe space in which the pregnant woman can resolve her hopes and fears. You can use this global storehouse of women's ideas to create your own unique homespun celebration, involving people who already have a special place in you and your child's life.

In the Wicca tradition, all life is seen as sacred, and a pregnant woman is honoured above all others as a personification of Mother Goddess. In the Silvery Tree ritual, the expectant mother stands inside a healing circle. This is blessed with 'holy water' (salt water left out and blessed on the night of the full moon). Sweet grass smudge sticks are burned to cleanse the circle, and evoke the protection of Vesta (the Roman God of the hearth and home). The pregnant woman is encouraged to explore her fears and concerns, so she is ready and prepared for childbirth. Prayers and blessings are made that she will have a quick and safe delivery, and a gift of sweet meal, oats and honey is given to the earth, as a thanksgiving for the gift of newborn life. Afterwards, people prepare and share a feast together to celebrate the woman's birth into motherhood.

In China, the older generations follow the custom of *tsue shen* or 'hastening delivery.' The maternal grandmother sends a parcel of new baby clothes to her daughter about one month before the baby is due to be born. This parcel includes a white cloth, which the daughter uses to wrap the baby infant in, as a gesture of continuity and love extending through the family.

In the Bengal celebration of *swad* (taste or longing), a lunch party is given in the ninth month to symbolize the pregnant woman's abundance. She is given gifts to show all her needs are fulfilled, her hands are hennaed, and her hair decorated with flowers. She receives a platter holding a little of all the foods on the table, symbolizing that she will want and lack for nothing as she enters childbirth. She takes the first mouthful of food, which includes a pinch of everything, and a conch shell is blown to show that she is delivered into the universe's protection.

In the Native American tradition, friends and family make a necklace of beads. Each person contributes and blesses an individual bead, which is then strung onto a single thread to make a complete necklace. The expectant mother is given this gift before childbirth, so she can draw strength and support from the combined strength of the blessings held within the beads as she goes into labour.

In the USA, a circle of friends may make a patchwork quilt together. Friends and family donate different pieces of fabric that they then sew into a quilt for the newborn baby to use. This quilt is created by a community of people with love, goodwill and laughter with everyone having an important role to play in the mother and child's lives.

You might ask friends and family to contribute items to make a birth book for your unborn child. You could fill this with anything relevant and important to you, such as your scan images, dried flowers and leaves collected from special times, photographs, pictures and words that give you joy, courage and inspiration, reaffirming the bonds connecting you to the people whom you love.

## The unfolding heart

One of the most beautiful gifts that you can give yourself is time; to be present and connected to your heart space. This simple act of being will soon be something that you savour and treasure on rare occasions. Never again taken for granted. Yet now, there is enough time to be alone.

There is a profound beauty in becoming truly comfortable in your own skin; to be conscious of the person you were, are now, and may yet become. In finding peace in solitude, you will become increasingly aware of the divine presence of love and wisdom flowing inside you – greater than the sum of your individual flesh and bones. As you realign yourself to your heart energy, you will begin to unravel long-standing contradictions in your life story. You become more receptive to honouring your creativity and intuition, bowing to the superior wisdom of the heart, to build an honest and compassionate relationship with your child.

## CONNECTING TO THE HEART'S ESSENCE

Sit down in a warm, comfortable space and close your eyes. Allow your breath to soften, relax and deepen. Become aware of your body's contact with the earth and feel safe and grounded. As you breathe slowly down into your belly, feel the warmth of your breath gently melt and dissolve any strain or tension that you are holding within you. Rest your palms on your chest over your heart. Become aware of warmth, heat, energy, light, or any other sensations in your heart space. Rest with quiet attention.

As you breathe in and out, follow the wave of energy rising up from the base of your spine into your heart space. As your breath flows, imagine your heart is cast awash in a sea of clear emerald green – an intense soft greenness that glows like a vibrant meadow of young grass after a rain shower in springtime – bright, tender and alive. As your breath connects with your heart, this soft luminosity radiates outward, bathing every cell and particle of your body in clear green, brilliant light.

Hug your unborn baby close to you with your breath, nurturing them within this healing stream of love, warmth and peace. Slide one palm down to rest on your belly over your baby, while your other hand remains on your heart. Feel your energy moving between your heart and your child. Now let your arms relax down on either side of your body, with your palms facing up to the sky.

Take a couple of moments to rest before you open your eyes. Then sit quietly for a few moments and feel the wellspring of love rising toward your child.

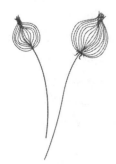

# GETTING READY
# FOR CHILDBIRTH

*'A hundred things may be explained, a thousand told, but one thing only should you grasp. Know one thing and everything is freed. Remain within your inner nature, your awareness.'*
**Padmasambhava**

Childbirth is a dance of creation between life and death. The act of giving birth is to manifest life out of the divine flow of energy running through the universe. However, the actual process of labour may not strike you as particularly sublime, involving bodily mess, discomfort, pain and exertion. It is the ultimate test of facing the unknown element of your humanity. As a mother-to-be, you cannot run away from the inevitable reality of birthing your baby. Yet, there is immense potential to transform the raw ingredients of childbirth into a source of higher consciousness, clarity and insight. To engage your heart and step through the gateway of labour, to get to know another side of yourself that you've never seen before. So when labour draws you out to your edges, you are ready to follow and truly witness this miracle of new life rising inside you.

So now you are on a mission to prepare your mind and heart for this incredible rite of passage. Labour and childbirth will drop you into the intensity of surviving on the edge of 'normality,' as your body functions under extreme conditions. You can guide your mind to embrace these extraordinary circumstances, expanding your usual range of perceptions, so you are ready and able to fully experience your own birth as a mother, as well as that of your child.

## Taking initial steps to prepare

Childbirth may be the most epic, gruelling and transformative experience that you ever have to live through. Whatever anyone says to the contrary. It tends to be extremely hard work, spread over many hours. Requiring copious amounts of resolve, confidence, stamina and endurance. You are achieving the metaphorical equivalent of climbing Mount Everest without oxygen. You are a heroine! Whatever way you look at your birthing adventure.

Your body already knows and can tell you how to do this. Your innate birthing wisdom will carry every cell and muscle in your body along in a current of labour, when the time is right. You cannot intellectualize this, even though you may complete and attempt to follow a detailed birth plan.

Labour will not necessarily wait for you to light the rose-scented candles at the point of delivery, regardless of whether your rational mind tells you to do this. And does any of the detail really matter when you face childbirth with your heart wide open?

Childbirth is a profound opportunity to touch the divine inside you as you participate in the miracle of creating new life. To step beyond your normal perception of reality, holding your mortal body in space and time. To see what you are truly made of when you surrender, let go of your resistance, and step into an unfamiliar experience. Moving far beyond your usual reference points of existence. To be present, sentient and engaged in labour, breath after breath, moment by moment, as life arrives with the passage of birth.

## Knowing your birthing parameters

You have the reassurance of giving birth, safe in the knowledge that contemporary medical expertise has drastically reduced the probability that either you or your baby will come to any harm. We are blessed to live in a world where we can give birth within secure parameters, with clear medical procedures in place to manage every conceivable complication that might arise. Yet the truth remains that even with all the help in the world, you are still the only person who can, and will, give birth to this tiny human being inside you. This is your experience alone. So while you may receive medical help during delivery, only you can trust and follow what your body is telling you to do.

You will want to explore the different birthing choices available to you. You can then make any necessary arrangements to ensure that these are in place sooner rather than later, so when labour arrives, you are ready to greet it. Your mind wants to be secure, confident and comfortable; sure about how and where you are going to give birth if possible. You can then divert all your mental energy inward to support your body, without worrying about the external logistics of how you want to do this.

Much of the flavour of your labour evolves around how far you trust your innate capacity to give birth and survive. You never know, you may even enjoy it! Women's bodies have understood how to do this, long before hospitals were invented. Rediscover this source of primordial wisdom buried inside you, so you remain grounded and confident of your own innate capacity to birth your baby as labour starts and progresses. Sure, it may not always go to plan – in fact, plan for it not to go to plan. Yet you can still encourage the mind to feel anchored and in touch with your heart, without getting caught up or distracted by worries, fears and anxieties about the direct impact of labour's passage through your body.

## Using your creativity

You might like to make a symbolic gift for your unborn child, making them something tangible to mark their arrival in the world. This creative process can open up your heart, reminding you to notice beauty, depth and colour in moments passing. You may feel a little self-conscious when you appraise your efforts, aware of the shortfall between what you want to create, and the object that actually arises out of your thoughts. Use your hands and heart to create a gift of love. This act of creativity can expand your parameters and

---

**SETTING OUT YOUR LABOUR SCENE**

You may want to think about the practicalities of labour within a birth plan. This will help to clarify your feelings about what is going to happen before it does. You may want to have a birthing experience full of flowers, essential oils, music, birth ball and a birthing pool. Helping your body along by practicing different birthing positions.

Know what visual objects you want to have near you, that hold special meaning for you. You can draw upon these to find solace, strength and courage, to give you greater resilience as labour progresses. You also need to ensure that that your birthing partner understands and respects your wishes, especially in relation to non-essential medical intervention. So you are confident of holding the course of your labour steady, even if you have to change direction.

---

WHAT CAN I MAKE?

Your first gift to your child is something unique. It expresses your love and appreciation of them when they are born. You might sew a baby blanket, design a patchwork quilt, or produce a painting, poem, papier-mâché model, or bowl. Or else start a birth book of pregnancy, adding memories, photos and words as your child grows up. You could then give it to them on their 18th birthday as they stand on the threshold of young adulthood. You might be concerned that your artwork isn't good enough, and has a certain schoolgirl feel to it! Don't worry too much. Your child won't judge your gift on whether you show artistic talent like Picasso. The most important thing is that you are making them something special. This is more than enough.

sense of possibilities. Setting you free you from self-imposed limitations. If nothing else, making something special for your child promotes authenticity, letting you laugh, and dissolve inhibitions, as you find different ways to express your innermost feelings and aspirations.

You can then direct your creativity into the process of labour and childbirth. Transforming your experience of labour and childbirth from a mere physiological function, into an act of self-transformation and discovery. The art of giving birth can be a spiritual exploration, an affirmation of life rising within you. Your spirit is rekindled as the small human being within you is born.

## Becoming at one with the birthing process

Your body is the perfect vehicle for your child's birth. Yet your mind still has doubts and fears about whether you are going to be able to do this. To enjoy labour, the mind needs to jump on board, working in synergy with your body. Otherwise, your mental faculties may try to revolt against the unfamiliarity of childbirth, reacting against labour sensations, because they don't recognize or know them, as part of your usual spectrum of experience. It doesn't matter if you have given birth before. You still need to give your mind the right message. And then constantly reaffirm that you can and will enjoy this incredible process of labour. So you are comfortable and confident about your role on the birthing stage.

You can mentally prepare for birth by visualizing how your body is going to manage and adapt through each stage of childbirth: starting with your initial contractions; then active labour as your uterus contracts and pushes your baby's head onto your dilating cervix; transition, as your baby moves through your pelvis into the birthing canal; and finally the delivery of your baby into your arms. As you develop a positive mental imprint of the entire labour process, your mind learns to recognize and follow this cue when the reality kicks in. You are building up a mental reservoir of empathy, resolve and determination to draw into your body, when you actually need to steer a clear passage through childbirth.

## Building up birthing resolve

This is your birth, no one else's. Labour is a hard and often arduous process. So you need to develop mental stamina and the determination to engage in it, from start to finish. Start preparing your mind and body so you're ready to face childbirth, even if you don't yet know how it's going to be for you.

The Sanskrit word *Tapas* comes from the verb 'to burn.' It is our inner fire of resolve that heats our intentions, transforming them into action. Through developing strength and effort, we burn away doubt, inconsistency and hesitation. Reinforcing and firing up our courage to keep on going. Even when you lose track of where you're heading. You might forget the ultimate point of what labour is all about – oh yes, you're giving birth to a baby – especially when you're in the thick of it. Yet by developing mental focus and concentration, you can see straight ahead to the end goal of giving birth without faltering.

You don't need to be blind to the challenges of labour that lie between you and your baby's delivery. It may be that the birth is difficult, and you need to change tack through labour, moving far away from your original birth plan. The warmth of *Tapas* generates inner certainty, enabling you to remain consistent in your focus and resolve. So if your mind wants to worry and tells you to expect the worst, don't falter in your intention to face labour's reality. Shrug off doubts and fears, and continue heading on in the right direction, fuelled by the inner heat of positive intention.

## Drawing a picture of labour

Throughout your nine months of pregnancy, you can draw pictures and images to reflect your individual, changing impressions of childbirth. You may like to build up a portfolio of artwork that represents your hopes and fears about giving birth. This is a starting point to explore your psyche in relation to becoming a mother and having a baby. Your pictures may reveal a lot more than you know about who you are: some of which you are already aware, along with other things that come to light. They may show you where you need to grow and heal to be able to fully participate in your birthing process. To connect to the fact that motherhood is actually happening to you. It doesn't matter whether you believe you can draw or are creative. Stickmen are fine! What matters most is to unlock seeds of genuine self-expression, rather than caring about the final outcome. So be prepared to put yourself on the line, expose your vulnerability, and know your true feelings.

Moving beyond words, express your childbirth in colour, shapes and symbols to see how your mind conjures up a self-image of yourself in the midst of this reality. Knowledge and words will not birth your baby alone. So birth art empowers your mind and body to participate in labour and childbirth as a living form of creativity.

## BRINGING BIRTH INTO MIND

Take yourself into a state of deep relaxation, removing external distractions, and making your body comfortable. As you breathe into your abdomen, let the muscles of your pelvis soften and release. This stream of oxygen-rich breath nourishes you and your baby, enabling your body to work more efficiently through the birthing process. Feel your life force flowing into your uterus, heart and lungs, as all your body's systems gear themselves up to work at optimum efficiency. Be ready to enter labour and deliver your baby into your arms.

Become aware of your baby's physical presence. Feel the weight and movement of your baby inside your womb. Ask them to place themselves into an optimum birthing position. Your baby's head is resting deep down in your pelvis. When your uterus starts to contract, they will slip quickly and easily down your birthing canal toward delivery. As you go into labour, you feel calm, alert and know you can meet the rising tide of contractions.

As you move deeper into labour, give your body permission to have regular and rhythmic powerful contractions, allowing your uterus to open, and your baby to be born. You can hold your mind steady and responsive, steering your way through the rising tide of birthing energy, rather than getting pulled sideways into mental panic, or trying to resist or prevent what is happening. Take hold of your mind, by returning your focus to your breath. See if you can concentrate on your breath flowing through you, more than on any thoughts whirring around inside your head. As you move into active labour, come back to your breath again and again to help you to move beyond the intensity of your contractions into measured relaxation. There is no reason to fight the peaks and troughs of your body's energy that are working to give birth to your baby. Instead let your mind rest in a place of refuge and fill up your mental reserves, so you are coping with the physical edges of each contraction as this comes and passes.

You are confident, at ease, settling into a steady birthing rhythm that enables you to relax and restore equilibrium in the space in-between contractions. You are delighted to be having strong, regular uterine contractions as these encourage your baby to press down on and open your dilating cervix. You are starting to move toward the delivery stage. Your baby is exactly the right shape and size to slide easily through your pelvis. You feel deeply connected to your child as you work together to enable them to have a safe passage through and out of your body.

You are now pushing your baby out into the world. You feel the muscles and tissues of your perineum and vagina easily stretching to allow your baby to comfortably leave your body. Your body's muscles spring effortlessly back into their original shape after you finish giving birth. At the point of delivery, you can feel your baby's head at the opening of your vagina. You breathe deeply, present, alert and engaged with your baby. Welcoming them into your life. You are ready to reach out and hold your baby close to you as you arrive in motherhood.

Imagine your birthing process before it happens. In visualizing a positive birthing experience, your subconscious mind starts to create an upbeat impression of how labour is going to be. Start using birth visualization as regularly as you can, adding in as much detail, authenticity and emotion as you can muster. While useful to practise often and early on in pregnancy, it doesn't matter if you only start in your last few days before birth. It is the sincerity of the intention and focus that gives strength and meaning to a birth visualization. Reaffirm internal cues that your body will recognize and respond to effectively. So when the contractions kick off, your mind is ready to prompt your body to follow a strong, positive image of giving birth. Now your body knows where to go.

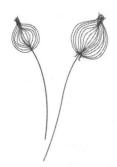

# OPENING YOUR SPIRIT
# TO CHILDBIRTH

*'You shall not separate your being, and the rest, but merge the ocean*
*within the drop, the drop within the ocean.*
**Tibetan Buddhist teaching**

What changes inside when you open your heart to welcome and embrace your entire birthing experience, in whatever shape or form it comes? Decide to enjoy it. The sky will not fall down on your head, no matter what anyone tells you. Try to be wholehearted and cultivate mental discipline to be present, turning your attention inward if labour gets difficult. Remain relaxed, focused and positive, resting in the stillness of your heart.

This is a basic living truth. When you listen to your heart's wisdom, you uncover joy, courage, insight and consciousness to live out the physical intensity of labour and childbirth, whatever you may have to face. It's that simple. Allow your mind to dwell in your heart's centre. Then the subconscious thoughts, emotions and sensations that push and pull you about can loosen their grip on your psyche.

You may never live in a constant state of awakened fearlessness. Instead, you can develop your capacity to trust and cope with whatever labour and childbirth throws at you. If this is an excruciating 24 hours of sheer hard work, along with medical intervention (planned or otherwise), to arrive at your baby's delivery, it's worth it! You can transcend any initial reluctance about childbirth, manifested as negative thoughts, sensations and emotions about what labour is to be – your inner cries for help and rescue. Align your mind to your heart's drumroll of courage, and be ready to face your human vulnerability in the experience of giving birth. All it takes is resolve to keep on going, doing the best you can, without giving up.

You don't have to define your life in relation to the fears, doubts and anxieties that wash over you. As you face labour, these nebulous clouds can easily threaten to weigh down your positive resolution. Let them go. Allow yourself to be conscious and present, led through labour under the guidance of a higher wisdom and truth. Listen to your spirit calling you to action. Your birthing experience will then be a reflection of a deeper spiritual intention to engage with and participate in labour, however it unfolds.

## Making friends with fear

Your due date is drawing close. Your thoughts may want to revert back to all the scary things that could go wrong between now and the end of childbirth. The very nature of childbirth *is* unpredictable, a tightrope between life and death. You have to relinquish autonomy and immediate control over what is happening, stepping into the unknown. You don't know how it's going to feel like when you do this, even if you have already given birth before. That was then, this is now. Each time will be a unique experience, without any precedence. You can't decide how labour manifests in your body. However, you can choose to take any wayward thoughts in a positive direction that is constructive to your birthing process.

So it may be worth contemplating your imaginary worst possible childbirth scenarios, so you can try to look at these worries and anxieties straight on. Invite them to tea, and find out the names of your individual fears and concerns: who and what they are and where they are going. It helps to articulate what is blocking your energy and holding you back, however trivial this may be. When you put a name to wavering angst, you can do something proactive to dissolve its latent strength and power over you.

The stronger the inner light that you shine on your murky thoughts, the clearer you can see them, exactly as they are. When you break small pieces off a large lump of clay, it starts to crumble and eventually turns to dust. So try to identify, then accept your fears in the open light of conscious awareness. And they will start to shift to become a more manageable concept, something that has no real existence, except in a future that has yet to come.

Be gentle on yourself when you wobble, yet vigorous in shaping a more positive train of birthing thoughts. Be vigilant! Don't let your mind get away with conjuring up scaremongering sessions that catch you unaware. You can regain genuine initiative, as you influence your fears into proportion. Identify the antidotes you need – courage, trust, confidence and determination – along with relevant coping strategies that act as a support to them. Shake up your fears and look at them from a different perspective, generating spontaneity, humour and a sense of the absurd. Your fears can have only as much potency as you choose to give them. Allow yourself to face what they are, without shuddering. Then throw them away so you are free to respond to labour with presence.

### The different shapes of labour's dark clouds

There is so much that could happen during labour and childbirth. The mind is adept at casting different shapes of negativity to hang your worries on. Remember these are not a reality, but just an abstract idea. And even if you spent the next few months dwelling on the worst of your fears, it still doesn't mean they are any more or less likely to happen. However, if you get too busy thinking about a possible disaster that may never strike, you might miss finding labour's elation and ecstasy within you, because your mind is travelling in the opposite direction.

The shape of birthing fear may fall into different archetypes:

**Failure**

You worry that you won't rise to the occasion, and don't have a natural aptitude for childbirth. In fact you're scared you'll be demanding an epidural within the first ten minutes of having contractions.

**Death**

The only certainty in being human is that we are born, and then we die. The probability that labour will bring death in its wake is remote, regardless of any morbid fascination you carry about this. Yet you still may think about this happening, even though the odds are highly stacked against this.

**Self-consciousness**

Labour comes with an unspoken dress code of removing your clothes, or at least stripping down to a scanty hospital gown. So although we all have much the same body as the next woman, two legs, two arms, one vagina, one head and the rest of it, we still feel embarrassed about showing this in full view of our audience.

**A sense of violation**

You dread intrusive medical examination or intervention. Anything that makes you feel your body is not being treated with respect, or as your own property. You worry that medical professionals will take over your birth, and start running your body's labour show.

**Losing control**

You hate the idea of sharing such an intimate moment with strangers who may not always be empathic or receptive to your emotional needs. You may not instinctively like these people or want them to share your birthing space, let alone trust them to act as you would like them to.

**Pain**

You can't ignore the association of labour with pain, even though you're trying hard not to call it this. The sensation of labour is intense, as your cervix opens by up to 10cm so you can push your baby out of your body.

**Parenthood**

Forget worrying about the labour process. Your major panic is about how you and your partner will cope with this baby after giving birth. You just don't feel you are parent material, or ready to put this to the test.

## Accepting the nature of uncertainty

We live in a results-orientated world that likes to measure success in terms of tangible achievements. We tend to view the amount of time and effort that we put into things, as a sort of insurance policy against failure; a self-made guarantee that our life will remain on track. To have a definite expectation of any labour outcome ignores the vital truth that life isn't always predictable. It's impossible to know what's going to happen before it does. So it follows that you can't know how your baby's birth will manifest for you. And having an idea about it doesn't count.

You don't want to be stuck in labour looking for an emergency stop button because things are turning out differently than you planned them. Your experience of childbirth may well be nothing like what you thought it would be. Your body in labour is not programmed to follow a birth plan. And do you really want it to? When it comes to the final push of getting your baby out of your body, you may feel very differently about how you want this to be done than you did a couple of weeks, days or hours ago. So you may as well happily embrace the joyful uncertainty of not knowing from start to finish. You can't control you body's birthing process. Except to trust that everything is unfolding as it is meant to. Your body knows what it needs to do, now let your mind listen to and follow it.

## Let your birthing partner speak for you

Your birthing partner is your advocate who reaffirms what you need. This person is there to support and protect you from external distractions and pressure, freeing you up to concentrate on your primary task of giving birth.

Your birth partner can help things along, by creating a safe and quiet haven around you, without unnecessary intrusion, noise and distraction. Of course, a hospital environment runs on its own terms, but you are still

---

**TRUSTING YOUR BIRTHING CAPACITY**

If you know that your body is a perfect instrument of childbirth, then what is there to fear and worry about? The affirmation of 'I can' is the perfect vehicle of a clear birthing intention, infusing every cell, muscle and tissue of your mind and body, as you prepare to give birth. As the tide of labour rises, the immediate relevance of the outside world recedes. This is when you create a safe, protective bubble of birthing energy around you that places you firmly at the helm.

Do you truly believe in your personal capacity to give birth? Do you actually feel this with deep certainty inside you? By assimilating labour and childbirth with your intuitive wisdom, you can give birth, and allow the miracle of life to transform you. You are an amazing, incredible woman who is going to give birth to another human being! This is the ultimate expression of your humanity. Have faith and the confidence to go with labour's flow, rather than shutting your mind or heart down to this unique life experience.

---

entitled to give birth in a safe environment where you are comfortable, secure, and able to get on with it, as your body knows best, without unnecessary interference.

It follows that if you want to have a go at having a natural birth, your birthing partner needs to know and understand your wishes, so they can actively help and support you to realize them. They will be able to articulate your birthing preferences to medical professionals, so there is no confusion about the direction you want labour to take. If you are then offered medical intervention, your birthing partner is ready to step in and see if this is strictly necessary, or whether you want it or not.

You need to feel you can speak to your birthing partner about anything on your mind without reservations, so they can empathize, listen and act in your best interests. You want to trust them to keep you on track if your resolve falters, without jumping into panic mode at the first instance.

Choose your birthing partner wisely, as a friend who gives unconditional support, kindness, comfort and reassurance. They can really make the difference between having a positive and joyful birthing experience, or one that you'd rather not repeat again in a hurry.

## Standing your ground and knowing when to bend

Your role in labour is to give birth. Everyone else, your birthing partner, midwives and medical staff, are there to support you to do this. It follows that you don't need to compromise on your birthing preferences, as long as you and your baby are healthy, safe and doing fine.

A natural approach to childbirth may clash with the medical culture of some hospitals, especially with constraints on maternity resources. Medical staff can be under immense professional pressure to meet birthing quotas, to get women to give birth as quickly and efficiently as possible with minimal fuss. In practice this can mean that you are offered additional pain relief on a routine basis, to help things along. You have a right to choose whether you want to accept this or not, when it's not a matter of an emergency procedure.

Make a clear decision about what you want to do, yet know that you are free to change your mind, whenever you want to.

Although your body is made for birthing, you will still have to tolerate some degree of discomfort. This may develop into a level of pain, fatigue and exhaustion, which can become counter-productive to you and your baby's health. At which point, be realistic about what you hope and expect. If you have been in labour for a long time and it's getting too much, you can always accept some medical intervention. Only you will know if this is the right decision or not; it is your choice alone, made in the best interests of you and your baby.

There is a delicate line between being flexible to change, and knowing when to stand your ground. We live in a society that likes a perfect happy ending. Having a natural birth isn't synonymous with this. At the end of labour, the only thing that is important is that you are holding your baby in your arms. And you are both intact. So don't dig your heels in, at your own expense. You are the creator of this happy ending, something that you sculpt from your individual interpretation of events unfolding. Following the natural birth option through from start to finish just may not be feasible, or compatible with this. So don't just follow it through on principle, when you don't want to. Your humanity and meaningful participation are the crucial factors in having a positive labour experience. So make sure you are mindful of this, whatever route you take. It is your birth alone, regardless of the precise details of how you ultimately get there.

## Changing your mind

Give yourself the freedom to be present and see what happens, without fixating on your expectations. Enjoy your labour as it is. You don't yet know, nobody knows, how you will find and respond to the unique essence of your childbirth.

You may follow an alternative path from what you originally planned. Sometimes a change of direction needs to made urgently. Remember that you can't always control how things turn out. Soften any residue of disappointment or regret. The ultimate point is that you are going to meet your baby. And as a mother, this is what counts above all else.

Accept how you experience each stage of labour. Feel a steady stream of compassion and kindness pouring through you. When you are in contact with the wellspring of love rising inside your heart, your energy keeps flowing. Your mind is fluid, and doesn't get stranded within a state of turmoil, pain and congestion. A warrior in the middle of battle doesn't stop fighting when things get difficult. They just change tactics or direction, gaining fresh perspective on the situation. Focus your attention on finding comfort and ease in your birthing body and mind. So you can see clearly ahead to where you are going.

## You and your baby are in this together

You can't give birth without involving your baby. You are in it together. Your baby is as an integral part of your pregnant body. And you are the centre of your baby's small universe. Your baby redefines this boundary through childbirth, as they expose their vulnerability to the world outside. This is a profound journey of separation, through togetherness. You can reassure your baby as they prepare to move out of the comfort and safety of your womb into unfamiliar territory, to draw independent breath. Giving unconditional love to your child lets them know that you are always there for them.

Your child soaks up the ambience around you, growing in the subtle vibration of your thoughts and feelings. When you communicate with your baby in and out of the womb, you create a living bond of love, trust and nurture between you. Your child can be deeply reassured and soothed by the nurturing sounds, movement and feeling tone of your emotions. You show them that you care deeply about them before birth. This builds the loving foundation of your relationship as mother and child that slowly develops into maturity, after they are born.

## Finding the source of love

At the centre of life is love. When you breathe love into giving birth, you infuse your mind with authenticity and compassion, even as you struggle with the physical reality, the intensity, body fluid, mess, effort and toil of pushing a baby out of your body. Your labour becomes a spiritual process, more than a merely physiological function of your pregnant body, within the confines of a hospital room. Your mind is conscious, connected to a source of divinity that ignites you and your baby's lives. As you open your heart to birthing your baby with spirit, you transform the bare essence of giving birth into something sacred, profound and universal. You are both a witness and a participant in the endless cycle of life and death.

You have a wonderful capacity to give unconditional love and compassion. This is the essence of your humanity. Your baby opens up a living gateway into your heart, through their presence in your life. You are held in your birth partner's love, the fond wishes of friends and family, and the goodwill of all the Buddhas and Bodhisattvas on this planet. You are carried on a carpet of blessings that can sustain you, as you prepare to give birth to your baby.

### THE OPENING LOTUS OF YOUR HEART

Allow your attention to rest in your heart centre. Visualize a pure white lotus flower, or a white rose in bud. As you breathe in, this bud slowly unfurls, each petal opening. As you breathe out, relax and rest deeply in your heart. Your breath touches your heart space.

See each petal of this exquisite flower unfolding with each breath. As your breath flows, feel love flowing through your heart and body, as you accept and give your mind, body and spirit over to the task of birthing your baby.

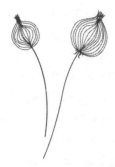

# SWIMMING DOWN THE
# RIVER OF CHILDBIRTH

*'Peace immediately follows the giving up of expectations.'*
The Bhagavad Gita

When water runs along a course, it flows over and around any obstacle that lies in its path. Like water, childbirth has its own natural flow of energy. As you go into labour, your body unleashes powerful waves of uterine contractions to help you to push your baby out of your body. So follow your body's rhythm without reservations. Remove any physical or emotional obstacles in your way. This is not a time to react with mental analysis or inhibition, unless this helps you to birth your baby. You have everything to gain when you let go, and let in the tide of new motherhood.

You are swimming along labour's currents. As your mind is swept along by the fierce intensity of contractions, it can be easy to forget the ultimate cause of why this is actually happening to you. Don't lose sight of the baby inside you, waiting to be born. You may start to forget the point of remaining in a state of mental equanimity, focus, resolve and sanity, as you begin to tire of the arduous demands of giving birth. Of the growing relentless intensity that starts to increase, exactly when you want to hit a pause button. Come back to the basis of your humanity – your breath, contact with the earth, the love you hold inside your heart. Remember that you are giving birth to your baby.

Being in labour is unlike anything else in your past archives of experience. Each birth is different, unique, special and a miracle. You will feel labour inside you differently each and every time you give birth, even if you have done this before. So be prepared to dissolve your thoughts, let go, and swim in the dynamic flow of labour as it draws you toward childbirth, in its own unique nature and time.

Hold onto the props you need to keep buoyant and afloat: your breath, your partner's fingers, voice, shouting, moving about, using a birthing pool, chanting, massage. You can't run away from your shadow as the contractions course through you. And you can't swim against this stream of labour without causing your body to tense and shut down. So reaffirm your intention to open, soften, stretch, relax, centre and swim freely and strongly toward the birth of your baby. Your child is waiting for you.

## Opening the doors into active labour

Sooner or later, you will enter into a parallel world of childbirth, in which normal parameters of adult life no longer apply. Your mind and body are consumed by the effort of birthing your baby. When you reach this stage of active labour, your contractions become stronger and closer together. You can no longer contain the torrential river of energy coursing through your body. Trust yourself to keep going, contraction after contraction. Try to encourage yourself to stay calm and motivated, keeping the end goal of your baby's birth in mind; letting go of anything that flies in the face of your positive resolve.

This is the reality of childbirth. Your mind may want to define your contractions with a corresponding flurry of emotions, in an attempt to control them. Your natural human response may be to let your mind jump into panic mode, to start ringing loud alarm bells with the label of 'PAIN' written on them. Fair enough! Strong labour contractions are not for the faint-hearted, and are rarely defined as fun. You have possibly been in labour for several hours, valiantly coping with increasing fatigue and discomfort, with the end nowhere yet in sight. And the reality of coping with pain is understandably pushing it up to the forefront of what you notice about your birthing experience.

Keep carrying on and on. You have everything to gain! Your body is working overtime to enable your contractions to become more intense and frequent, a sure sign that your cervix is starting to dilate and open. You'll then be ready to move into the final stages of delivering your baby. Everything is going to happen as it is meant to. Believe you are nearly there, and soon you will be!

## The scent of self-confidence

Your subconscious mind may whisper negative thoughts through labour such as: 'I'm not really enjoying this' or 'Help! Get me out of here!' You don't want to hear this commentary, but it's set on repeat mode, running inside your mind. Drawing you into the quicksand of doubt. It's frustrating, but true! Yet labour doesn't have to be a self-fulfilling prophecy of doom. Don't give up, just because a part of you wants to. Stop tuning into your ego's blatantly unhelpful suggestions, and concentrate on the other side of your psyche; the part of you that wants to create and participate in a positive birthing experience.

You are able to do this! The starting point is to believe with every cell in your body that you are birthing your baby. Trust in your heart's wisdom and feel the affirmation rising up within you. You are a strong, resilient and positive person; get to know the depths of these qualities as a reflex during your labour process, and when you arrive in motherhood. The paradox is, that as you accept your vulnerability and acknowledge your jelly legs, you become uninhibited, powerful and free. This is the gateway to your true nature: uncovering new reserves of inner strength, resolve and courage to carry forward with you.

## Finding the spirit of labour

Listen to your heart. Allow your spirit to lead you through the physical intensity of giving birth. Create a clear mental image of your baby being born, reaching out to follow this internal map through labour's physical course. Concentrate on meeting each one of your contractions with determination, courage, strength and patience. They will not last forever, however easy it is to forget this.

This isn't a place of conditioned and weathered responses, of half-heartedly going through the motions of labour in action and ignoring what your body really wants and needs you to do. Shout, chant, sing, groan, swear and dance with all your being. Do whatever it takes to open up your body and heart, and get this baby born. Let labour happen! You are merging your mind and body in the deeper flow of life force that aligns you to the universe. To know and live this is a gift, connecting you to all living things.

Allow childbirth to unfurl inside you like the petals of a flower opening. Your body is dilating, contraction after contraction, until your labour comes into full bloom. Expand your consciousness as your baby is drawn into life. You are both giving and receiving life. Connect to the universal rhythm of life flowing in, around and through you. Embrace your higher self's wisdom as this guides you toward the birth of your baby and yourself as a mother.

## Stepping outside your comfort zone

Most of us like to live firmly within our comfort zone; we prefer life to be easy, predictable and operate within clear outlines. We rarely choose to come close to our edges, preferring to stay within the circumference of what we know, like and can easily assimilate into our lives. We don't want to struggle to integrate too many difficult experiences into daily normality; it disrupts

CREATING INTENTION THROUGH WORDS

There are many beautiful words to help you to create positive intention. You could explore one of many yogic mantras on love, compassion, or overcoming inner obstacles. Are there any words or phrases that ignite your consciousness, as you contemplate giving birth? After spending time exploring your fears about childbirth, now generate the qualities that you need to cross over the river of labour.

Your intention is the basis of your own individual mantra. Each time you speak, whisper or silently repeat these words with sincerity, you build up their potential to manifest within you, taking you into a place of refuge. Hang onto these words fiercely, softly, drawing them deep down into your birthing body.

What is your deepest hope in giving birth? What affirmation will hold you steady as labour takes place within you? What phrase can you create to remind you to stay on track when you're in the midst of contractions? Your mantra carries your spirit through labour, empowering you to lodge and plant the vibration of these words inside your heart. As you say and reaffirm words with meaning, you wash your mind and body in their healing strength and intention. This inner jewel glistens within you, lighting up your path through labour when things get difficult. All it takes is one thought to glow strongly, to show your mind and body where to follow.

our status quo. We may fleetingly glimpse over the precipice from time to time, and then quickly move back into our secure, stable and safe definition of reality.

There is nothing wrong with this. It's understandable, often sensible. Why go out looking for a real-life dragon, when you can find one in a story book. However, it does mean that if we never get to know the outer edge of this invisible boundary, we decrease our capacity to fully engage in life with all its possibilities. To enrich our lives, by exploring the unknown. We place limitations on our potential existence, confining ourselves to evolve around what we should do, rather than what we can do when the sky is our limit. We take the life we know for granted, always playing it safe and predictable. And we are seldom moved to witness the extraordinary.

You may be someone who does delight in exploring the raw, extraordinary essence of our humanity. You like to live on the edges when the barriers are down. Your life is punctuated by moments of great elation, as you discover new depths of experience to explore. Throwing off the safety blanket, whenever opportunity arises. Whether that is by diving into an ice-cold sea, training your mind to reach new heights of achievement, or overcoming great personal obstacles to learn new skills. One thing is for sure, you are seldom bored, finding new depths of colour and awareness within conventional patterns of living.

Yet, there will still be times when we feel small, dull and insecure. We then have no choice, but to face our personal struggles against a sense of inadequacy. When we confront that we may not be able to do something, at least not in the way we want to, we come up against ourselves. You already know where your doubts and fears reside, sometimes in the most unlikely places. So the challenge is to step up to the edge of your comfort zone, and then go beyond. This is the raw truth of facing yourself with honesty, opening up the living space in which you tend to operate. Expanding out the circumference of your life, you increase your physical and mental capacity to live the extraordinary, and receive greater abundance.

MANAGING DISCOMFORT YOU CAN'T IGNORE

You can help yourself to feel more comfortable and at ease with an array of holistic or clinical pain-management techniques. Do your research well before labour starts, so you know what's on offer and can remember how it works. Yet be aware that you still need to be present in your body to give birth. You can't escape or run away from this. Even with a flotilla of pain relief at your disposal.

You don't control labour, although it can control you. So don't try to contain and hold it within an acceptable level of sensation. There is no right or wrong birthing sensation. You can only experience childbirth as it is. Sometimes the only thing you can do is to accept things as they happen. Your body in labour is constantly changing. And your mind may soon define your current sensations as something else. So trust and find inspiration that you are moving in the right direction toward your baby's birth.

In labour, you are going to live through extremely challenging circumstances one way or another. And once you are in this place, there is no going back. Your mind and body are going through massive emotional and physiological changes to birth your baby. Not always comfortable, but never dull. While you cannot necessarily change labour's shape evolving, you can guide your mind to manage and perceive this, to make it into a potentially sublime experience. Taking into account that labour is happening, whether you like it or not. There is no get-out clause. And by its very nature, it is extraordinary. It requires an extreme shift in your normal definition of living, so that your wonderful baby can be born. And you can be fully engaged in this process. Accept that it can only happen if you make that quantum leap, and believe in miracles.

## Understanding contractions

Become curious and attentive about the nature of your contractions. Observe how they start to build, peak and subside like a wave rolling into shore. See if you can breathe and move through this strong wave of energy, rising up

### RIDING WAVES

Imagine you are sitting on a beach watching the sea of your labour stretching out in front of you. Observe the waves of birthing energy crashing into shore, as they simultaneously move through your body. Follow your body over the peaks and troughs of each wave of contractions. Sink into relaxation as you rest before the next set takes shape. Find deep stillness in the lull between each wave. There is a space here to fill up with strength, courage and resolve, to gather your resources so you can ride over the rising peaks of the next wave, moving freely and easily over the crest of its intensity and back down into peace. Your mind and body can calmly move with the tide of childbirth taking you toward the birth of your baby.

and over its peak and resting in the space between. As the next one starts, go with the flow of sensation again, and again. Notice how your contractions are constantly changing in shape and form, each one different from the last. Your labour is an evolving process that moves your body forward, opening to allow the passage of life through you.

Watch as your mind defines your birthing experience. You have the mental discipline to move fluidly beneath your surface impressions of labour's sensations. Past your habitual response to pain as something that is unacceptable and downright unpleasant. To be present to the incredible nature of childbirth as you find it. Seeing it afresh as each moment arises, letting go of preconceptions, and coming to terms with the reality of being in labour. You can't escape from this situation, so look closely at how your mind moves through sensation, and what this tells you about its nature. So you can accept and create the perspective that you need and want to have.

## Surviving the peaks and troughs of contractions

As another set of contractions builds up within you, you may believe you are at the limits of your endurance. You simply cannot take any more of this. Your mind gets tossed about, drawing you out to the extremes of what you can tolerate, pushing you over the edge into an abyss of pain and fear. You don't want another contraction! Yet, as much as you think, 'I can't do this', know that your body is still doing it, regardless of whatever you choose to say about it. Your intuitive mind is coping remarkably well, releasing birthing hormones through your body to stimulate and strengthen your contractions. Birth is happening!

We spend so much time and energy trying to run away from ourselves. Falling under the spell of shadowy monsters of inner turbulence, we fail to notice that our immediate feelings are already moving, shifting and changing into something else. When we look closely at our mind, we can see our emotions aren't solid or tangible. They are fluid, flowing like water in different directions. Yet we still allow ourselves to believe in the solid shape of negativity made up of mental illusions. We put ourselves down into a quagmire of doubt, fear, angst and contradiction, even when this hurts us.

So, as you stand tottering on the edge of your mental precipice, you can look down into the unfathomable depths of human experience. What are

---

**FINDING YOUR WARRIOR SPIRIT!**

So here you are facing a strong current of labour rising within you. This is tremendous! Inspire yourself to be a warrior, rising up to the great challenge that lies ahead. So yes, you are anxious, reluctant and half-hearted about stepping forward to embrace childbirth with open arms. Create personal cues to ignite and reaffirm your determination, courage and resolve. Motivating you to follow the onward surge of your body's energy into unknown territory. You cannot dream and float your way through this. This is no time to get lost. Open up to wholeheartedly participate in one of the most incredible and sublime life experiences you may ever have. Let life arrive within you. Live each moment of childbirth, one step at a time. Let yourself glow and shine as your inner light guides and helps you to find your own unique way through labour's pitfalls.

---

you capable of facing? You are surviving, even when you think you can't manage to hold the intensity of labour's contractions inside you. Stretch out your edges, expand your inner core of strength and courage, and rediscover the essence of who you are, and can be.

## Catching hold of the reins

When horses were wild and spent their days roaming free on the plains, their natural instinct was to run away from predators in the vicinity. So when you ride a domestic horse, one of the basic rules is to keep hold of the reins to stop the horse from bolting away out of control, especially when you don't want it to. Otherwise, you literally give the horse a 'free rein' to follow its natural tendencies, to gallop off in any direction it chooses.

The mind is like a wild horse. When left to its own devices, the ego can quickly lead us off and away into a kaleidoscope of random thoughts, sensations and feelings seemingly unrelated to each other, and without much sense to them. When things are difficult, before we even realize what's happening, our thoughts are traveling off on a downward spiral of doom-like negativity. So what will you do if your mind decides it doesn't like what's happening, and tries to flee away from the situation? Given that labour is highly intense, and often excruciating, it's likely this could happen. You need to be alert, engaged and ready to catch the mind. Especially when you are nervous and anxious about this unfamiliar territory. Get ready to guide your mental responses, so you don't automatically resist and try to push childbirth away from you as far as possible.

If your mind tries to run away like a wild horse, you will get pulled in different directions. Many of which may lead you close to panic, fear, anxiety and distress. Losing control just isn't worth it. You might start to perceive childbirth as something painful and terrifying that you have to fight against. When the mind loses control, you're in danger of giving up autonomy; rendering yourself powerless to cope with labour as it comes. You then have no other choice but to let it happen to you. And it's much harder to enjoy

**FINDING INNER LIGHT**

You are made of light. Imagine a golden orb of light shining above the crown of your head. This radiant light is overflowing, pouring down into your skull, your body. Filling every muscle, bone, cell and tissue within you with clear luminosity. Nothing can extinguish this healing light's resonance streaming through you.

As your heart beats, this clear golden luminosity spreads, radiates out into the space beyond and around your physical body. It cleanses your mind, lifting you up to connect with your higher self and consciousness. Meeting sharp edges of sensation, this healing light softens and melts rough, jagged points, as your body labours to give birth.

Connect to the source of your inner light. Find union. You can dissolve the physical intensity of what you are feeling in this infinite source of divinity flowing from the universe through you.

anything that comes with this precondition; you're literally making it much tougher on yourself.

So what if your rational mind wants to hide under the stairs until it's all over. This isn't the point! You still have to live through labour in progress, to get your baby born. And the only person in the world who can do this is you. While all the other people in the world may encourage and support you, you are the one who is giving birth. Think about it. Your labouring body is already dealing with massive physiological upheaval, so why complicate matters further and lose confidence in your body's natural capacity to get on with it?

Take hold of the reins of your mind, and direct all your resources into giving birth with clear positive intention. You are responsible for holding your mind steady. It's up to you to remain open, flexible and receptive to

the situation. You can do this! You *are* doing this, with courage, resolve
and strength. Steer yourself firmly toward feeling the deep, warm glow of
satisfaction in directing every cell of your being, into the effort of birthing
your baby.

You have the potential to transform childbirth into a profound rite of
passage, more remarkable than you ever dreamed it could be. To witness and
experience labour as sublime ecstasy and transformation, as you discover
your innate ability to manifest your baby's new life on the planet.

### Your inner voice

Your voice is a vital link that connects the intense energy unleashed inside
your labouring body to the reality of processing this experience inside you.
Your use of sound in labour is a channel of self-expression, helping you to
deliver your baby from your womb into the world outside.

At some point during labour, you may communicate beyond words,
finding a spectrum of instinctive sounds deep within you. Your mind may
struggle to hold onto the social norms of small talk when your body is
consumed by birthing your baby. Non-verbal communication can express
your feelings far more aptly than the thread of conversation. Let your
labouring body finds its voice and speak clearly to you. It is liberating to let
go of the social etiquette of conversation, without minding whether you raise
an eyebrow or two!

Your voice can then become a meditative tool, guiding and focusing your
mind through the extremities of giving birth. As your body births your
baby, you create a symphony of birthing energy that clearly resonates in
your mind. You can follow this path of sound and vibration into a state of
heightened concentration and relaxation.

### Breathing your way through childbirth

One of the simplest ways to harness your mind through labour is to follow
the rhythm and movement of your breath through your body. Your breath

flows down inside you, giving you an anchor that leads you inward to your baby. Each breath connects you to your baby, providing them with a rich supply of oxygen in their blood, helping your labour to progress more efficiently, bonding you together as you both move toward the point of your meeting. Your breath is the energetic fuel that helps labour along, helping to relax your body so it hurts less. Breathe deeply and regularly into your body. As you breathe into your belly, feel your breath flowing smoothly through you, warming, opening, touching your womb and your baby. As you exhale, dissolve stress, melting tension in the healing warmth of the life force that holds you. Each new breath revitalizes you and your baby, connecting you to each other and the cycle of life. Use your breath to stabilize and clear your mind, to steer a clear course through childbirth.

## If you lose your breath

Our breath rate is changing all the time. When we exercise hard, our breath tone quickens as we need to take shorter, shallow breaths. The same happens when we are under mental stress or exertion. Our thoughts become agitated, we become restless and wound-up, and the nature of our breath tone changes to reflect this. So the regular, even breath of a relaxed person stands in contrast to the shallow, uneven breath tone of a tense person who is hot and bothered.

The good news is that it is easy to change the quality of our breath tone. In doing so, we also change our state of mind to reflect this. So during labour, if you need to cultivate mental equilibrium, or else raise energy levels, find this quality within your breath tone, and your mind will follow. Start by deepening your exhalation, gently lengthening the time it takes you to breathe out. Feel your breath flowing out of your body. Let go of any strain or agitation. Cultivate spaciousness within you. Light up dark soft, velvety space inside your body with your breath's energy.

Consciously breathe out over the rising peak of contractions, arriving back down again into your resting zone. As you concentrate on your breath flowing, your mind disengages from the immediate sensation of each contraction. You start relaxing and expanding the rhythm of your breath, and your mind quiets into calmness. This is wonderful news. Your parasympathetic system is now free to release feel-good endorphins; something it can't do while adrenalin and stress are charging around your body. You actively make your body feel better when you breathe reassurance to you and your baby. Finding support and comfort in each breath.

Keep your breath flowing regularly in synergy with your contractions as they rise and subside. You are then consciously nurturing your mind and body, helping your baby to cope with the extremities of labour and delivery, breathing a clear path through each contraction, until you both reach the other side of childbirth.

## Your connection with the earth

Your centre of gravity is your foundation, helping you to feel centred, comfortable and grounded. Feel the contact of your body in labour with the earth's surface. Exhale and direct your breath into your pelvis. Breathe into your roots, and draw life energy into your core.

If you disconnect from your breath, you become displaced from the earth's energy flowing within you, impeding the natural rhythm of labour. On the other hand, you support your mind and your body by being present to, and engaged in, each breath.

Connect to the earth through conscious awareness of your breath. Breathe out fully, deeply, giving yourself to the earth's protection. Let your breath melt any tiredness, strain, anxiety and fatigue. You are part of the earth, and the earth is a part of you. The sun makes the plants grow to become food that nourishes you. The clouds give rain, giving you water to quench your thirst. The spaciousness you create inside your body echoes the sky stretching out above you. Your lungs are filled with fresh air around you. Your life is a microcosm of the earth, a reflection of the whole. Breathe out blessings for this life you live, your baby's life, and the new mothering life that you are moving toward.

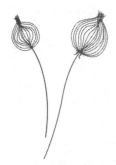

# ARRIVING OUT ON
# THE OTHER SIDE

*'The seeds of the plants are blown about by wind until they reach
the place where they will grow best . . .'*
**Okute, Teton Sioux**

You have followed your body into labour, and survived to tell the tale. The reality of giving birth at the edges of sensation is an assault upon your senses. And can leave you feeling traumatized, exposed and insecure, beaten-up in mind and body to some degree. No matter how or where you gave birth. You need space and time afterwards to assimilate your experience of childbirth, so that you come to terms with it, heal any residual hurt, and move on.

## The aftermath – processing childbirth

The voice of our inner critic often delights in making us feel less than perfect. It articulates doubts that we didn't do enough, and highlights what went 'wrong' in our lives. Be aware! Your self-judgment may try to reduce the sublime profundity of childbirth into a limiting definition that reduces your experience. It wasn't this or that, or somehow you failed in giving birth. You didn't! Your baby is born. And that was the only vital thing necessary to get done. Life is as it is, and labour happens as it does. The baseline is that you lived through the miracle of giving birth, and became a mother.

You can't change the details of how you gave birth. But you can honestly acknowledge and accept how you feel about this experience. Talking to someone who was present and whom you trust, can help you to make the transition into conscious mothering. There is little point in trying to ignore or hide difficult, conflicting emotions and sensations about labour, out of a misplaced fear that these will somehow define you as a new mother. You can't say you succeeded in labour or not because it isn't a test, and what can you compare it with, except your own body's experience. And what is the point of that? You delivered your baby into the world, however they arrived. Express and reflect on what labour was for you, so you are emotionally free to get to know your baby.

Shift the tone of your personal perspective on your labour, to find a wavelength of resolution inside you. Look around you. Notice how far you have come, and everything that you have to celebrate. The fact is that you pushed yourself to the limits of your existence, and gave birth to a new human life. This is the work of a heroine!

## The gift of healing and recovery

Your body has just survived a massive influx of birthing hormones, the dilation of your cervix by up to 10cm, and the physical delivery of your baby out of your body by whatever means was possible, into a separate life outside of your womb. All of which is definitely not a part of your body's normal range of experience. So now in the aftermath, you need to rest and recuperate. Only you can create this healing space. Allow time to slow down, and find quietness and peace around you. You can look after your newborn baby at a steady pace, without rushing to keep up with the impact of change rippling across your life. Catch hold of each moment of time, and be present to it. This is a time to focus on getting to know your baby as a unique individual, and yourself as a mother, within your new family structure.

After a peak experience comes a trough. This is where you fill up your reserves. You don't want to deplete your internal energy and strength, burning out before you reach the end of the first month of motherhood. Your beautiful little baby is utterly dependent on you to meet their entire spectrum of needs. It's up to you to therefore decide to cultivate a strong sense of vitality, health and wellbeing, to cope and thrive with the challenges of looking after them around the clock. Your baby does not need you to become a mothering wreck of nervous exhaustion, illness and irritability. So take responsibility, setting a maternal speed and pace that you can keep up with, and also enjoy.

You may feel that you will never again be the same woman that you were before birth. Celebrate your courage, bravery and effort, alongside any sadness or pain at a difficult or traumatic birth. Start filling up the holes, leveling out your emotional landscape until you feel ready to let go and move on. When you believe that you are managing, things start to get better; your body will respond and follow in the path of your healing energy.

Your baby is likely to be pretty exhausted by the physical ordeal of labour, along with the new stimulus of arriving on planet earth. They will probably be quite content to spend much of their first few days sleeping and quietly getting used to their new status quo. You can enjoy the relative calm, finding respite, quietness and space with them, until they fully arrive and start to make their presence more actively known to you. Grab any chance you are given to rest and catch up with yourself. You may not get this time to catch up on sleep again for a while, until your baby accepts the elusive concept that night equals bedtime and not playtime.

There is no looking back now, no dress rehearsal to practice in. You just have to get on with being a mother as best as you can. Look after yourself each day alongside your baby, making active choices to sustain a healthy balance of equilibrium and wellbeing across your life. So you nurture your child in the clear, calm and loving reflection of your mothering spirit.

## Understanding the baby blues

After your baby is born, the display of interested concern showered on you during pregnancy tends to evaporate. Instead, the spotlight of attention is turned onto your baby. You may largely become invisible. Your needs and

---

**SETTING THE SCENE**

In China, the new mother makes an offering of incense and sweetmeats to the earth goddess who helped to conceive her baby. After childbirth, the mother enters a 'sitting' month in which she stays at home in a warm bed, to rest and recuperate with her newborn child. She is relieved of normal chores and responsibilities within the household, so that she can heal and recover from childbirth. It is said that this is a 'cold stage', so the mother needs to build up internal heat. She is given warming nutritious broths, and avoids cold or raw food, to help rebuild her strength and vitality. At the end of the month, her family and friends hold a birth party to celebrate the mother's return to a full life again, and to welcome the newborn baby.

---

feelings are ignored or forgotten, as you revert back to being just you, albeit with a larger waistline than nine months ago.

The bubble of upbeat euphoria that surrounded your baby's birth tends to pop after the third or fourth day. This coincides with a dramatic drop in your progesterone and estrogen hormones, to the levels they were at before pregnancy. Many women feel weepy, tired and pretty flat, as the mind struggles to keep up with the physiological adjustments of the body in this postpartum phase of life. Hold tight! The baby blues are a natural dip of human emotions; a precursor of the joy, hope and wonder that will also come, as you walk a fragile line between the highs and lows of motherhood.

## Postnatal Illness (Depression)

Human happiness is a variable emotion, standing in sharp contrast to sorrow. It may be that you struggle with the more serious medical condition of postnatal illness (also known as postnatal depression). This can affect up to one in ten women after childbirth, drawing them into a downward spiral of negativity. It requires active help from family, friends and professionals. The warning signs include tiredness, irritability, lack of interest in sex, depression, guilt, anxiety, feeling low and not being able to cope.

Most of us will feel some of these things as we struggle to integrate a small baby into our adult lives, while looking after them around the clock. This unfamiliar territory of new motherhood soon brings strong, buried emotions and thoughts up to the mental surface. Once there, they overflow into our new reality, overwhelming our attempts to have a positive response to the maternal challenges we face. Sometimes the world sits heavily on our shoulders and life feels like a burden. Yet already your emotions are changing and moving elsewhere.

## Accepting help

What can you do to help yourself to adapt to motherhood? To smooth out the teething problems and emotional hiccups, which can easily develop into a tempest in a teacup – especially when left to brew. Understand where your fault lines lie, so you can actively support your mental and physical recovery after childbirth. Don't be shy or proud to ask for help on your own terms. Ask friends to prepare a meal, keep home visits short and don't be motivated by a sense of misplaced duty. Instead, draw clear boundaries around your family space, so that you relax and rest, while sharing the joy of having a newborn life in your midst.

As a mother, you need to be able to put your baby first, above all other priorities. To do this, you need to be able to keep the rest of life running on smooth tracks, so it doesn't derail every time you turn away to change your baby's nappy (diaper). Don't think you have to carry everything on your shoulders, especially while you are adapting to motherhood. Share some of the weight. It is your prerogative to choose what you would like other people to carry for you so you can focus on your most important priority: learning to carry the weight of your baby with grace and ease.

Your time is no longer your own. You are living at the beck and call of your baby; anticipating their every need, often before they even express it. Jumping up to look after them upon demand. Yet you can still rest in the gaps between childcare activities, as you leap from one point to the next. Find space inside you, even when there is so little in your world outside.

### Moving on to the next stage

Come to terms with your birthing experience, with love, acceptance and understanding. The passage of birth exposes your own vulnerability, the essence of your mortality, even as you are witnessing your baby's life beginning. Appreciate how far you have come since the early days of your pregnancy. You have danced between life and death, holding your baby's life within your own. Your world is changing; it will never be the same as it was before.

Your heart is awakening, springing into motherhood. The boundless depths of love and compassion are rising up within you like a foundation,

### RECLAIMING INNER SPACE

Lie down in a quiet space and make sure you are warm and comfortable. Allow yourself to stretch out, your legs resting hip-width apart, your feet falling out to each side. Let your arms lie beside your body with the palms of your hands facing up. Gently lift each shoulder blade in turn, and release them down to the earth. Move your neck gently from side to side, allowing the muscles to lengthen, loosen and release. Your body is in contact with the earth. Become aware of the back of your skull, shoulders, arms, wrists, hands, spine, pelvis, backs of legs, ankles, feet and the spaces between. The force of gravity draws your body down to connect with the earth. Witness your breath as your body breathes.

Scan the entire length and breadth of your body, starting from the crown of your head and moving down toward your feet. Drawing your attention over each part of the body in turn. Cultivate expansion and warmth, allowing tension to dissolve away into the earth. Make a conscious decision to soften, lengthen, and relax each muscle, until your entire body enters a natural state of equilibrium and peace.

This is your body. Where are you resting now? Accept your feelings, whatever they are. Understand what you aspire to be, but are maybe not able to find yet. You only have this one moment; it is now. This is a time to be present, without doing, trying or effort. Lie resting, watching your breath moving, allowing deeper waves of relaxation to wash over you. Sometimes all you can do is let go of any pretence, and just be as you are.

spilling over into your child's life. Bridging the gap that we create between ourselves and all other things; to know our true nature through uncovering joy, contentment and peace inside us, and learning to reflect this outward into family life. We find we are part of the same universe as our baby, the world that gives us our life, and everyone else. Listen to the calling of motherhood, and follow this path leading you into a new cycle of spiritual renewal and growth.

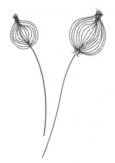

# GROWING INTO
# CONSCIOUS MOTHERING

*'To see a World in a grain of sand,*
*And a Heaven in a wild flower,*
*Hold Infinity in the palm of your hand,*
*And Eternity in an hour . . .'*
**William Blake, *Auguries of Innocence***

Your nine months of pregnancy have passed. You are now the mother of a beautiful baby. You have long anticipated this moment of your child being born, and how best to weave your adult life around their infant one. This is the ultimate time of change, when you take a giant step forward into the reality of motherhood.

You soon develop a maternal reflex for changing nappies (diapers), feeding and winding your baby and surviving on minimal sleep. And you effortlessly multitask beyond the requirements of any previous job: rocking your baby to sleep, preparing food, eating meals one-handed on the phone while tidying up with the other. Yet when you lift your head up from the intensity of mothering life, you may begin to see emotional cracks appearing on the outer veneer of your maternal ecstasy and bliss.

Yes, you are coping, well pretty much most of the time. Yet, there is also a growing sense of anticlimax. The excitement of pregnancy and childbirth

### KNOWING TRUE WISDOM

You can always gather up copious amounts of information and advice about the logistics of having a baby. This covers a startling range of viewpoints on child development: how to manage your infant's sleep pattern, play activities, feeding schedules and every minute detail of their tiny lives. You can fill buckets with external knowledge from experts and professionals, and form a measured, surface opinion. Yet this is so different from knowing the source of higher wisdom and insight that lies inside you. When you draw your mind inward and shine light on your heart, you become aware of what your child needs. Without anyone else telling you. Nobody else's opinion matters here. Listen to your own knowledge, truth and guidance.

Don't be complacent or make do with secondhand facts that sound impressive, but aren't found with discernment. Bring what you know into your heart to see whether it rings true. Transforming it into wisdom. Here, you'll find all the answers you need. This is the path of true understanding: self-inquiry or *Svadhyana* is to know the universe that lies inside. Anchoring your mothering experience in the pure light of your higher consciousness, guiding you to truth and wisdom. And you don't need any book, including this one, to tell you what this is!

soon fade into memory, and hanging out with your baby around-the-clock becomes second nature. Of course you love this little person. Yet it's hard to reconcile maternal devotion with the relentless, tedious and often exhausting nature of childcare. You are not the first woman to wonder if they are missing the whole point of motherhood. Even as you simultaneously catch your breath and fall in love with your child, all over again. If you are nodding your head in recognition, it's time to shape your daily mothering experience in the light of cultivating mindfulness, of what 'is.'

## Stepping outside the myth of perfection

Forget the fairytales. That you will suddenly become a 'better' or 'nicer' person now that you are as a mother. On the contrary, it might seem the opposite is happening. Looking after small babies and children, with their antisocial sleeping patterns, fussy feeding, wind problems and unreliable volume controls, is bound to rock your emotional boat. You can't buy a miracle cure to wipe away the internal suffering that comes from being human. And your mothering life with a young baby is no exception to the rule.

You may vow that you will never ever be a mean, grumpy mother, or shout and hiss at your baby, however fraught you are. And maybe you won't. We all hope to live in family paradise, sharing a plateau of domestic harmony and peace with our partners and children. Yet most of us are still trying to find our way here, even long after our children have grown up and left home.

So, while your newborn, tiny baby is adorable and gorgeous, your nerve endings may also be fraying, your resilience put under immense strain. And some days, it may all feel too much. You feel pulled in a hundred or more different directions, pushed to the absolute limit of your endurance. You could easily break into a thousand pieces of despair and frustration. In short, it's time to consider where you stand in all this. One minute, you take it all in your stride, and feel you've cracked it. The next, the thorns of motherhood get under your skin. You feel agitated, in turmoil, brooding with unhappiness and dissatisfaction. We all struggle to reconcile the double-edged sword of relative emotions, only able to appreciate joy and peace, through their polar opposites of negativity and pain.

Forget your aspirations of being a shining example of constant maternal happiness and serenity. Our children expose the rough edges of our psyche, revealing our emotional boundaries. Where we need to change and grow. Let go of the woman you once were, and get to know the mother that you are becoming. Shake up your perception of who and what you are, and can be, so motherhood is a comfortable fit, through all the stages of your children's lives.

## Accepting resistance

When you're on a maternal roll, your heart is content and expansive. You bask in the glow of your baby's presence. Yet at the same time as fiercely loving your baby, you may sometimes struggle to willingly be the sun in their galaxy. You clutch at your autonomy, hanging onto its shreds, before it dissolves under the impact of placing your baby at the centre. Maternal love takes you into the heart of your baby's universe, even as you struggle to orbit around them. You sometimes want to push your maternal responsibilities away. You crave space and freedom for a few hours, days, to do whatever you want, when you want. On a bad day, you may fail to carry out your parenting role with any heartfelt conviction, especially when your baby is unhappy, whiny and discontented. It's a bit of a shock to realize that while you love and cherish this shouting mass of humanity, it doesn't always translate into appreciation or enjoyment of their company.

It is likely that you will only adapt to looking after your baby after surviving some emotional hiccups along the way. For most of us, family life holds varying degrees of joy, wonder and satisfaction alongside chaos and frustration. Often we direct this in roundabout ways at ourselves, and manifest further impatience, irritation and angst. Yet we never give up looking for a stop and reflect button, so we can try to create a more sustainable version of happy families.

## Loosening maternal expectations

Your reserves of goodwill and patience can run very low with the relentless demands of managing fussy babies, older children squabbling and other minor catastrophes. To discover that someone has eaten your slice of cake saved for later, can trigger major domestic warfare, with emotions exploding like ammunition. You are likely to be operating on low levels of sleep as your baby keeps nocturnal hours – a form of political torture in some countries! And this may cloud your perspective. It is understandable to become doom-ridden, like a lonely troll living under a bridge.

When you accept that being a mother can jar your nerves, you don't have to pretend to be an imaginary figure of maternal bliss that you're not. You can be more resilient to your mental ebb and flow, taking responsibility for how you express your feelings. When family life is difficult, appreciate the things you are doing, rather than criticizing your current position.

So yes, you might have periodic moments when everything, even the toaster burning your toast, is out to get you. The background noise and commotion of new mothering life can overwhelm your senses, and your emotions slide into conflict mode. The sole purpose of having a baby is not to destroy you, even if you sometimes perceive it like this. Change the scenario, retreat and escape from the danger zone. Your mind is already moving on. Have hope in what the next tide brings.

## Emotional honesty

Navigating through new maternal territory unlocks strong thoughts and feelings, not always expected. Life changes, hormonal changes, the whole lot can make you feel vulnerable and extremely sensitive. Give yourself kindness *and* honesty. Look at the whole picture, treading gently, without fighting aspects about having a baby that you struggle to cherish or enjoy.

It may feel gratifying to play out certain feelings in your domestic soap opera. You try to provoke a reaction of sorts from your family audience, to balance the weight of your own suffering. Yet when the curtain falls and your emotions subside, where are you left? Still carrying the burden of your suffering. When we blindly follow our internal dialogue of thoughts or emotions, we are led away from the heart's wisdom, acting out a part that we may later regret. Even when we are justified in doing so – we did so want that last piece of chocolate cake! – we remain stranded from our heart's guidance, with the fractured pieces of our equanimity scattered around us.

Our emotional reaction often shows more about our inner state of balance than the actual situation that prompted it in the first place. Another time you won't even notice what provokes you so much now. You don't become a vampire by dressing up as Dracula occasionally, even though you may feel like one at the time. And your children definitely won't turn into holy figures when they act out the Nativity at Christmas. Observe your emotional barometer when you are drawn into strong outward projections. Step away from your internal dialogue. Observe your feelings, without always throwing yourself into the drama that they might suggest.

Anger doesn't need to translate into screeching fury and stamping feet, or sorrow into tears and anguish. You don't have to become a caricature of your feelings. Accept them without becoming them. When you are over the moon with joy, you don't need to act like a stereotype of happiness, hugging strangers in the grocery store to express your delight. Accept all of your emotions. Hold them lightly inside you, and then let them go.

You are constantly learning to adapt your actions to fit around your changing perspective. Trying to ensure that you don't act out of proportion, or lose emotional control of situations. At least that's the general idea, even if your emotions still spill out of the pot. Yet while you may feel like you're drowning in emotional soup at times, the mind is already moving on to another stimulus. It never remains fixed on any one thing for long. The current bubble of drama pops and evaporates. And soon you can't even

FINDING EQUILIBRIUM

When you next face a difficult situation with your child, observe how you are feeling inside your belly. Are you comfortable with what you find there? Accept whatever sensations you notice. They can't provoke a mutiny, or take over your life forever! The opposite! Allow your emotions to breathe and evaporate. By stuffing them back down inside you, they stagnate and mutate into mammoth proportions. It's no use saying that they aren't there, when they are, lurking inside.

So much depends on where you choose to put your attention. Use your breath to guide you to a deeper source of stillness and peace at your core, even as your feelings run loose around this. You don't gain lasting satisfaction in getting caught up in any one emotion for too long. So when you notice a tantrum stirring, let those feelings pass through you, then refresh your perspective and allow yourself to notice something else. Understanding your own nature helps you to change and to do things differently.

remember what all the fuss was about. More to the point, you just aren't feeling it anymore.

## Uncovering magic

Your senses interpret your life story. When you are floating in tiredness, come back to basics. Be attentive to what you see, feel, smell, hear and witness, and create a storehouse of wonder to last you a lifetime.

Our mind is kept so busy interpreting sensory stimuli, sending its findings back to our body that we are constantly building a picture of how we *think* our world is. This usually happens in the blink of eye, without us even noticing we're doing this. Slow down your sensory antennae to find beauty within the detail of your everyday experience. Notice life in its purest essence, as if for the very first time.

Redefine your relationship to the world around you. When you are attentive, you are aware of sensations as they actually arise in the present tense. You connect through your body to your environment, experiencing life as you are living it. As you slow down and take notice, the mind wakes up to reflect the miracle of joy, sorrow and beauty, inside and around you.

### Being receptive to authenticity

Accept your metamorphosis of self and identity in the wake of children. Self-understanding is the path to inner peace and happiness. To be authentic and receptive to whom you actually are, without pretence, self-torture, or delusion. Observe how you are constantly evolving into new ways of being, dropping old expectations. You are in perpetual evolution, a mother in progress. And what you are now will be different tomorrow, as you encompass new maternal horizons.

To recognize your strengths and weaknesses is a significant step toward living with love and compassion as a mother. Self-acceptance is to know what you are, not who you want to be, showing you where you are heading. You can't hang onto your old status quo and priorities. Only let your perception catch up with how things are now. To think that you are a certain type of mother, that 'I'm like this or that', is vastly different from knowing and living this truth in action.

## REDISCOVERING THE SENSES

Sit down in a place at home where you enjoy being. Allow your mind and body to relax and settle into stillness. Observe your surroundings as if you were seeing them for the first time. Notice the interplay of colours, the dance of light, the patterns of shadows upon objects around you. Observe your mental dialogue without following threads of conversations. Ignore internal voices telling you to get up and clean away any dust or dirt you notice on your sensory journey! This is about you, as you are now. Let your mind remain attentive, noticing what's around you. Accept your surroundings exactly as they are.

Shut your eyes. Become aware of different sensations on your skin: the texture of fabric, air, warmth or cold, and your breath. After a while, listen to the noises around you, a clock ticking, baby chatting, floor creaking, your body and breath. Now notice sounds outside, whatever they are, without wanting to change them. Hear each sound as unique.

Give yourself a few minutes to appreciate this moment. Now get up, stretch, and open your eyes again. Keep your gaze soft and focused on your immediate surroundings.

Take this exercise outside. You might look at just one thing in detail, or an entire landscape, either in an urban location or in nature. Notice what you see, hear, smell, taste and feel, through your living connection to the world around you. Witness the interplay of life upon your senses.

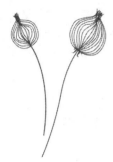

# OPENING UP
# A MOTHER'S MIND

'This world is nothing more than Beauty's chance to show Herself.
And what are we?
Nothing more than Beauty's chance to see Herself.
For if Beauty were not seeking Herself,
we would not exist.'

**Ghalib**

You can only look out of a window when the glass is clean and transparent. If the surface is dirty or obscure, it's difficult to see clearly. We view the world through the layers of our personality, the ego filtering our outer perception of life. Our sense of identity is a complex matrix, made up of how we think, behave and act, which is set on default mode. This cloak of mental conditioning may obscure the clarity of our perspective, directing thoughts and emotions into a repetitive, often rigid stream of consciousness. We remain so firmly entrenched in our psyche, that we are hardly aware of our personal nuances, let alone capable of changing them.

The glass cage of personality dictates the choices of our lives. Our perspective – how we choose to relate to the world – largely depends on how we look out from this prism. Our emotions may be bubbling up and over, before we have even noticed our thoughts rising. So our state of mind rarely reflects what we actually perceive in front of us. Instead our habitual reactions dictate our lives, like a chain of cause and effect. We seem unable to see and respond to the world with fresh eyes, except to repeat our past patterns of behaviour, regardless of context.

Yet now, after having a baby, there is the possibility of change. You are aboard a ship that is sailing swiftly out of harbor into new, uncharted waters. As your mind awakens into motherhood, you navigate through winds of change, able to find a new way of being. Pregnancy, birth and motherhood prompt you to reassess your sense of self and identity: your priorities, values, beliefs, culture, hopes and dreams. To find out what you have outgrown or want to revisit, in the fresh context of life with a child.

### Expanding perspective
We all have an idea of the person we believe ourselves to be. Yet sometimes, we are not so sure. We hold onto a self-image of 'I am this', believing in the illusion of a definite ego lasting forever. Until we come home inside ourselves, to experience a deeper stream of consciousness, a way out of this confusion. Our perspective expands then, beyond our deep-rooted

attachment to chasing daydreams around in circles. We grow to experience our true nature, beyond the limitations of repetitive thoughts, behaviours and feelings.

There will be afternoons, even days, when you would quite happily discard these new layers of motherhood. You would love to wear your old, comfortable identity again for a while, like putting on a pair of well-worn jeans. This feeling may sneak up on you when you're feeling under pressure to fit into your new role at the helm of a family. This might sound unduly negative, as you make your grand entrance into this gorgeous new world of babies. We start with genuine motivation to enjoy *and* do our mothering best at all times. Yet even when things are going pretty smoothly, there are still occasions when the milky bubble of maternal contentment pops. Don't feel guilty if your expectations then explode in your face!

Until you expand your inner perspective to adapt to your changing reality, you will only notice half the details in the picture that you are living. You can create a new landscape as a mother with a baby, different from anything known before. Adapt to change. This is a tremendous opportunity to find new clarity on old issues, to shake up and re-evaluate your old way of being.

## Accepting your emotional fabric

Become aware of your thoughts and emotions passing through you before you act on them. You may have good reason to feel angry, pissed off, irritable and frustrated by everything around you. This doesn't mean that you have to become the living personification of these feelings. We all tend to forget this in the heat of our emotions. Yet it is possible to feel things deeply, fully and passionately, without becoming them. You already know your danger points, when your feelings threaten to spiral and push you out of control. You can cope with whatever life with a baby throws at you, consciously responding with clear eyes to the situation at hand.

You start to observe and understand the mental reflexes of your mind; the internal dialogue that automatically switches on without you realizing. How your mind tries to leave you behind, like a runaway express train, before you're ready to jump on board.

So the starting point is to calmly notice the way in which you go about things. Find out who, and what you are: the types of behaviour, mindset, moods and reactions that you regularly manifest. Whether your mind is helping or hindering you. Become aware of situations in which you repeat the same old patterns from your past, so you can learn how to change your present. In moving through daily life with young children, notice your individual fault-lines, the flashpoints of internal stress and the chasms where you fall into an emotional void. You have a chance to catch hold of your mind and let the clouds pass overhead, your breath leading you into new space.

## Living in an imperfect world

We are often terrified by the slightest hint of imperfection and chaos brewing in our lives. It can contradict and threaten to pull down our efforts to create a linear life model, taking us in the direction of happiness, good fortune and

---

**TO LIVE BEYOND SELF-LIMITATIONS**

There is a deeper consciousness flowing beneath the surface appearance of who you believe yourself to be. When you know the true nature of your mind, you connect to an infinite horizon stretching out in front of you. Each day doesn't have to feel like an endless cycle of repetition, with constant strain to create a positive impression of your life. It holds a real possibility of fresh insight, change and wholeness. You don't have to live imprisoned inside the walls of your personality. Your mind can expand into spaciousness.

This is to find *Satya*, the absolute reality of who you actually are. The universal energy that flows through you, beneath the shifting impressions of emotions, thoughts and character traits projected outward into your life. Touching this source of divinity, benevolence, goodness with mindfulness, you arrive home. To the truth of who you know yourself to be, beyond limitations.

---

success. We work so hard to create the impression of stability. Here we are living in our home with all our possessions gathered around us. Never mind that we won't be able to take them with us after we die.

Smile more and complain less, especially when the world turns out differently from what you had hoped and expected. You can find comfort and ease in your place in the world, however it all turns out. You will miss what the universe is offering you if you're too intent on looking for something else. It is the quirks, strangeness and absurdities that make life so interesting, amusing and sublime. Celebrate differences with those around you. What does it matter that you look after your baby this way, and someone else does it that way? You didn't receive a blueprint of instructions at birth on how to do this living thing. And guess what? Neither did your baby. So enjoy finding your own personal path through the possibilities.

## Thought watching

Have you ever looked up at white clouds moving above you on a warm summer's afternoon? Or watched clouds scurrying through the darkened slate sky of a winter's day?

Look at your thoughts as they pass over the vast expanse of your mind. Notice ideas forming, words arising and the feelings and sensations that accompany them. See how they continuously change, let them go and become aware of your breath moving inside your body again. Until the next thought arises.

Your mind exists in a natural state of fluidity, constantly moving with the tide of breath from one thing to another. Observe your thoughts as they come and go, without attaching emotional meaning to the words they generate. See how your mind gets drawn in, falling into daydreams, make-believe scenarios and imaginary conversations. And then take your attention back to your breath again.

Your breath holds the mind's wandering attention. Now observe your thoughts passing across the backdrop of your awareness. As thoughts come and go, often with little reason, you can start understanding how the mind is. As long as there is breath, your mental activity will keep changing, appearing and fading. Sharpen your concentration to become mindful of whether your current mental projection has any relevance to what is actually in front of you. Then you can decide whether you want to give your attention, time and effort to a specific thought process.

## Transforming routine into something precious

There is an old Buddhist saying: 'Before awakening, chop wood, carry water. After awakening, chop wood, carry water.' On the surface, life appears the same. Yet as the mind wakes up, it becomes bright, spacious and expansive. Alert, attentive and able to appreciate the exquisite beauty of the shifting impressions it's living through. You are more able to create something extraordinary out of the normality you experience every day, bringing your life into light.

In the here and now, your days and nights are made up of countless routines to meet your baby's needs around the clock. The list of things you have to do each day may feel endless: clearing up, changing nappies (diapers), cooking meals, feeding, cleaning, housework, settling to sleep, household admin, going to work, laundry, cleaning up again and getting baby ready for bed, down to sharing the same games, nursery rhymes and songs again and again with your child. A vast proportion of your waking hours are mapped out before you even draw the curtains. Time gets swallowed up in cycles of repetition, without respite or spontaneity. Just the thought of another day can make you feel worn out and drained, half dead or at best, only just alive. And you haven't even got up yet.

No one wants to feel like this, of course not! There is boundless love for your baby floating around in your vicinity. And being objective, you know that the nurture you are giving them in these early months has immeasurable value. You also know that things will get easier as your baby grows older, independent and more robust.

You know that this stage passes all too quickly, and then you will look back and cherish these precious, fleeting memories of your children when they were so little. But all that is yet to come. Here and now it's still the same. At times, it is an uphill battle to maintain your sanity. Let alone to find contentment in the daily monotony of living around small, dependent children, within the confines of your domestic hemisphere.

Your capacity to maintain your motivation lies in charging your daily routines with positive emotional significance. When you are fully conscious of what you are doing, you arrive in each moment, rather than mechanically acting out a part. You become mindful, able to transform a mundane routine into a significant ritual that enriches you and your child's life with spirit and purpose. So while you are still doing the same thing on the surface, you appreciate and discover delight in what you are doing.

Your world may shrink to evolve around your baby, yet it can also expand to embrace the joy and delight of living with mindfulness. The external logistics of childcare might still remain the same. Yet with the mind focused and alert, you can live in the most frustrating or sterile of circumstances with spontaneity, wonder and appreciation. There isn't time to waste on

---

**THE JOY OF CONTENTMENT**

To experience contentment, or *Santosha*, is to appreciate whatever life has in store for you. Not because it happens like this or that, but because it is. Whether we find an experience easy, difficult, fun, horrible, something we want to repeat, or avoid like the plague, our mind interprets and defines it, influencing whether we see it as intrinsically good or bad. It all depends on the baseline we set ourselves. So one day, we laugh when we fall flat on our faces on a banana skin. The next time, we might sit down and cry, or hop up and down with rage. And yet, a week later we laugh again. Who knows! It makes no sense really.

When you're content, nothing matters as much. We use contentment as the common denominator of life's experiences, accepting what happens, when it happens. We live with greater ease, without minding too much when life slips up.

---

believing that things aren't good enough. Or else, getting stuck in regret, dissatisfaction, boredom and restlessness. Instead you decide to uncover each moment's potential, without loosing your hold on it. The mind settles into the present moment, and becomes calm and centred. And you are able to consciously develop the mothering experiences that you truly want to have.

## The art of appreciation

Slow down to absorb and appreciate your mothering role as you live it. It may sound gushy to go about your daily business wearing a sparkling tiara of emotional superlatives. Yet to live wholeheartedly without reservation and resistance, connects you to a bigger universe. It gives your life purpose beyond rushing through every 24 hours from start to finish.

Choose what you focus on each day, and find a genuine satisfaction in engaging your whole attention in ordinary experiences through the joys and sorrows of living with a child. Your state of mind reflects your relationships with yourself and others; now is your cue to raise the quality of these interactions. You are able to consciously change how you touch the universe. There is no need to look any further than where you are now.

Your concentration deepens. You start to discover an entire world in the microcosm of your life. Slowing down to become comfortable in your own skin. What else do you have in life, but the capacity to enjoy it?

## Opening the doors of simplicity

Listen to your spirit calling, and discover grace. Let the scent of beauty infuse your experience, revealing how life can be. Look at the natural world around you with fresh eyes. Wherever you are and whatever needs to get done, there is always time to stop, absorb and be aware; to see cobwebs of dew, the weight of raindrops poised to fall, the colour of earth tones, the light of dawn, the whisper of wind in the leaves, the warmth of sunshine and the seasons passing. Find pleasure in simple sensations: the coolness of water running over your fingers, the crispness of fresh linen, the burst of flavour in

### REACHING FOR THE SKY

Breathe in and let your arms float upward until your palms join each other over your head. Let your breath rise up the entire length of your body, from your feet up to the crown of your head. Imagine your spine lengthening as you draw your shoulder blades down toward each other, opening your chest and heart. Look up at the sky as you softly ease your spine into a gentle backbend spread out along each vertebra.

In Tibet, this *Asana* is called the 'sky diamond', which means opening your heart energy to the universe, while standing firmly on the earth's surface. Allow your entire body to breathe in expansion and space. Then let your arms float back down on either side, as you breathe out deeply.

fresh fruit, the sensuality of warm water in the bath. As you notice the rich detail of what is always there around you, you remove the source of your dislocation from the world. You heal the chasm between your thoughts and subsequent experiences. You create synergy between mind and body in the reflection of the puddles outside.

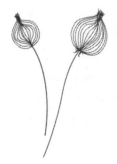

# AFFIRMATIONS OF MOTHERHOOD

*'All the happiness that exists arises from wishing joy for others,
and all the misery that exists arises from wishing for happiness
for oneself alone.'*
**Gendun Drup, First Dalai Lama**

What does it mean to you to be a mother? How do you want to fill this role each day? You possess so many wonderful gifts, talents and qualities to share with your children. Become conscious of what you value, of what is truly important to you. So you are aware of how best to inspire and encourage yourself when you don't know what else to do. You cannot possibly predict your children's personalities, but you can consciously guide them into adulthood. Set time aside to plant and renew affirmations within your family's life.

Each moment holds a choice – to believe in yourself as a mother, and trust in what you have to share with your children. Otherwise your maternal reality can be overshadowed by negative thoughts, criticisms and definitions, limited by what isn't right about it. Your heart alone opens and lights up your mothering path.

## Rebalancing the wheels of time

In the early days of mothering life, you chase minutes, seconds and hours, racing against a clock that you can't catch up with. Time doesn't serve us, but keeps us trapped in a relentless schedule of three-hourly feeds, preparing meals, playgroup sessions and diary entries. We all know the scenario of chasing after a few minutes in order to complete everything on our list before the parking ticket runs out. On the other hand, a rainy day at home with children can be excruciatingly slow, dragging by at a snail's pace. And then, we start to hop up and down, bursting with impatience, as our children struggle to keep up with our adult pace and priorities. We lose our deep-rooted human connection to the earth's rhythm.

While your children are still small, you are in a full-time mothering job, with only a few erratic moments available for you to snatch away. Your time is no longer your own, so you need to rethink about how to use it to feel alive and complete. It may not be possible nowadays to do all the things you'd like to do. You can't always choose to watch a movie from start to finish, read a chapter of a book, eat a meal while it's hot, or have a conversation without cutting it short. Yet we still have the capacity to thrive. We can follow the rise and fall of light from sunrise to sundown, aligning ourselves with seasonal change. We can listen and respect when the earth tells us it is time to eat, work, rest, play and sleep. There is always time each day to relax in, if you know where to find it.

Yesterday has gone, and tomorrow does not exist. Yet, now is the present. And here, there is enough time. There is always a list of things to do. But what really matters? Prioritize one or two things, and then leave the rest alone. Wake up without knowing what you are going to do by the end of the day. Enjoy whatever this is. Or, accept you may lose yourself in a cloud of adrenalin as you race over the finish line – and by then, you may not even remember what all the rush was about.

This stage of your children's lives is not going to last forever. And once over, it is gone. Enjoy what you can while you can, starting with how you choose to arrive at the end point. There isn't a reward waiting for you when you finish all the clearing up, cooking, caring for and entertaining of babies. So live your mothering life at a comfortable walking speed, with only occasional bursts of acceleration. Stop regularly and notice the world outside your family nucleus. And still, things will get done sooner or later.

## Practicing how to live at ease with your body

To feel comfortable as a mother, it helps to develop a strong, healthy relationship with your physical body. Physical yoga practice, or *Asana*, helps you to establish strong roots with the earth, and supports a positive lifestyle of mindfulness. Your human body is the tangible vehicle of consciousness. When you respect and look after the bodily structure of your flesh and bones, you can move with more comfort, ease and steadiness through your life. You develop strength, energy and resolve by planting your feet down firmly on the earth's surface. Allowing your heart to become present to the physical dimension of mothering, and making genuine contact with your children.

Through regular yoga practice or another bodywork discipline, you gently revitalize your body, releasing stress, strain and toxins. Also building a strong core of stability, strength and flexibility. You feel more relaxed and energized through dissolving congested, stagnant energy and tension. It can only lift your spirits, as you dissolve sources of accumulated stress, discomfort and pain held within you. Your life force and vitality flows more easily and freely in your body. You are able to direct your attention more fully, and engage with greater concentration in what you are doing, rather than living to barely survive.

## Stepping onto a yoga mat

You have a child. So you need to integrate them into your practice space. This may no longer be 'your' time; there is less quiet introspection. Yet you can still step onto your yoga mat when your baby is content and safely occupied, even if only achieved after putting on an episode from a DVD box set of cartoons, bought specifically for this purpose. Adapt your practice, exchanging silence for the richness of home life with your baby. Some days, it will be disjointed, as you stop and start again for the umpteenth time. Yet, your child will accept and absorb the ambience of your practice, as you dedicate time to breathe life into your spirit.

Your baby will get used to keeping themselves occupied for short periods, while you are in your practice space. And you will also become comfortable practicing with them in it. They may try and pull your attention toward them, join in or sabotage your plans, depending on where the wind is blowing. It is important for you and your child to learn to be together, yet self-sufficient; comfortable and content in your own separate spaces. They will know that you are still available and open to them, even when your attention is elsewhere.

Your children may not show any interest in your practice, beyond using your downward dog yoga pose as a bridge to crawl under. Yet you will make a subtle, positive impression on their mind and heart when you practise with diligence and integrity. Your child will only benefit from the renewed vitality and spirit that you take with you into the rest of the day, after you step off a yoga mat.

## Letting go into relaxation

How can you let go, when you don't know what you are holding on to? We all struggle to open up and embrace aspects of our lives with children. An inner rift develops between the golden dream we hang onto: how we want things to be, and the real-life version at ground level. If you secretly wish that things were different, you can build bridges between your two parallel universes. Use your dreams to draw your hidden fears and hopes out into the open. Your dreams may never materialize, but you can know the truth of living with a light and carefree heart. Regardless of what happens, be content with things, just the way they are. You are now stepping into light, and learning to inhabit your life.

The universe is changing in front of your eyes, even as you try to stand your ground. A stream flows along its natural course to join a river heading out to sea. When you are relaxed and content, your intuitive wisdom and heart energy are alert, conscious and guiding you toward your life purpose, whatever that is. Yet your ego tries to fight what is outsides its own jurisdiction, trying to control the unpredictable nature of other people, things and time. So you create conflict, dissension and division between your mind and its surroundings.

So what? Life can surprise you and shake you out of complacency. Surely that is the point! To surrender and find joy in whatever it brings. To find grace and ease moving with the flow of your life's energy, rather than against it. To become comfortable, as you accept and soften the mental barricades built up out of fears, doubts and insecurities. To breathe out deeply through difficult moments and dissolve the tension you hold inside. Each moment can only happen once in a lifetime! Smile and accept whatever each day brings, and welcome the unexpected into your life.

Each day may provoke sensations of discord, pain and displeasure, all of which pass sooner or later. And you get through the flashpoints of stress and chaos, maybe feeling fragile, but more or less intact. You are still here at the end of each day, living proof! When you are mindful and accepting of experiences as they come and go, your mothering life gets easier and more satisfying. You are transforming your inner response to what happens next into an adventure of discovery. Learning to enjoy the passage of time, day in and day out with a small baby, taking this understanding with you.

## The sanctuary of inner peace

Looking after your baby and family can over-stimulate your senses, stretching your mind and body so tautly that your nerve endings hum. Cultivate awareness of an expansive, boundless presence of peace within you. The pace of life with a newborn baby paradoxically seems to veer between extreme slowness and constant rushing to keep up with your baby's need for love, nurture and care. This is before you even turn to look at everything else that also matters and needs your attention. Being a mother commands a large proportion of your attention and energy. It is tiring to look after a baby or small child without respite. Especially when your body is screaming out for some sleep and time of its own. Soothe and replenish your nerve endings, so you are able to care for your baby wholeheartedly, without resistance.

You only need a few moments to find sanctuary. On the bus, waiting in line at the grocery-store checkout, folding endless piles of laundry, driving home. In this inner space of stillness, you are aligned to your heart, intuition and creativity. The world shines and reflects inside you again. You feel deeply, complete, content and whole, regardless of the superficial dramas of mothering life. Able to understand and listen to your children's needs and desires from your heart centre.

### RESTING IN YOUR LIFE FORCE

Vigorously rub the palms of your hands together and place them over your eyes. Allow any tiredness to melt and drain away. Stroke the palms of your hands over your head releasing tension. Brush your hands over your face and feel the warmth radiating out and relaxing each muscle. Draw tiny circles around your temples, your eyes and underneath your jaw line, and anywhere else that you need to dissolve tension and generate healing.

Massage the back of your neck along the occiput ridge at the base of your skull, using enough pressure to iron out any knots or tender points. Stroke out stagnant energy along the tops of your shoulders, down each arm and shake it out through your hands.

Brush your hands down the front of your body and legs, to the feet. Reach behind your back and rub your kidneys on either side at the base of the spine. Rest your palms on the back of your pelvis, around the sacrum. Feel the warmth and heat of your hands easing away achiness, tiredness, strain.

Feel love deep within you as you lay your palms onto your body, anywhere that is empty and drained. Supporting your body with the healing energy of your life force.

## Replenishment

Are you looking after yourself as well as everyone else in your family?
Do you ignore the vacuuming, laundry, dirty saucepans in the sink and
all the rest of it when your baby is napping, and sit down and rest too? You
want to stay on top of your life. There may be other children, relatives, pets,
work, all shouting for attention before you even try to fit yourself into your
living equation. So fill up as well, before you start running on empty.

If you've made an apple tart waiting to be shared out, everybody would
get a portion in your vicinity. Some people would receive a big slice, others
more meagre, but a slice nevertheless. Soon you would have none left to give
to yourself. And so you would go hungry. How often do you save something
back to fill yourself up with? Or you always make do with the leftover
crumbs at the bottom of the pie dish? You don't need to mutate into Mr.
Greedy, and gobble up everyone else's share of the attention and care that
you have to give. But you deserve and need to receive adequate nourishment
and care as well.

You will only be able to sustain a high level of nurture, when you
remember to give yourself something back, at least sometimes. You know
this simple truth already, even if you frequently ignore the messages that
your mind and body are screaming at you. To truly give the best to your
children, you need to be in a strong, positive state of mind to guide them.
There is no other way around this. When you look after yourself as a way
of life, you will be able to enjoy being the mother that you want to be.

If you are making an emergency crash landing, you place the oxygen
mask over your own head first, before turning to your children. This same
principle applies throughout your mothering life. Look at yourself first and
how you truly are, so you know how to be a contented mother with happy
children. This is not selfishness. It is self-preservation. Learning to develop
your self-worth and esteem, so that you have more to give.

The impact of neglecting your own needs will slowly creep up on you.
You believe you are managing to survive on meagre rations of sunshine,

food, exercise and relaxation. You are always waiting until later to catch your breath, let alone to consciously manage to breathe in the air around you, to connect with your life force. You live as if you were already half-dead, using up your reserves of energy, vitality and spirit without filling yourself up again. You cannot carry on like this without becoming a martyr, a victim, or turning into a boring old misery guts. Make a proactive commitment to creating wellbeing and equilibrium across all dimensions of your life. Not tomorrow, right now!

Feel the place you are at: the degrees of your tiredness, fatigue and exhaustion. Soothe and nourish your senses as fully as you can – through long hot baths with oils, candles, music, dimming the lights in the evening, letting your nerve endings find peace. A simple hug, the touch of a hand, a gentle back or foot massage, is balm to frayed emotions. Gently nurture your sensuality, grounding your energy and drawing up fresh vitality into your mind and body. Grab moments to deepen your reserves of inner strength and resilience. Start to arrive back into your body after childbirth and know yourself as the mother you now are and the one you want to be.

Before you reach the limits of your endurance, reconnect to an inner state of balance and equilibrium. Take responsibility and jolt your mind into finding out what it takes to feel on top of things, rather than sinking under them. You can hold all the pieces of your life with ease and grace.

### COMING INTO DEEP RELAXATION

When tiredness is endless, you have no more to give and start grinding to a standstill. Stop and rest. It doesn't matter what else you need to do afterwards. Stop for a few moments. Lie on your back with your eyes shut. As you breathe out, feel yourself being held by the earth beneath you. With each exhalation, let your body sink into stillness, letting go of tension, tiredness and all the rough edges.

Gently lift each shoulder blade in turn and replant them down. The palms of your hands on each side of your body are turned upward, facing the sky. Place your legs hip-width apart, feet turning outward. Allow your neck to soften and lengthen. Now become aware of the entire vehicle of your body resting quietly on the earth's surface.

As you rest deeply, your senses slowly settle into stillness. Observe the sensation of your breath moving naturally within you. Your breath lengthens and softens, washing and cleansing your body, dissolving tiredness in its wake. Soak up the healing power of deep relaxation. Lie still, resting your mind and body for up to ten minutes or longer, knowing that when you return back to what you need to do next, you will be rejuvenated.

Revitalize yourself with breath. Feel the residue of fatigue drain away into the earth. As you breathe in, feel pure life energy refresh your mind and body. Notice the touch of air moving across your face, the sensation of fabric on your skin, and let your senses reconnect with the world outside. Gently move your fingers and toes from side to side. Stretch out your arms over your head. Then bend your knees and roll over on to your right side. Lie there quietly still, with your eyes shut. Hug yourself.

Lastly, push yourself up again to a sitting position. Sit calmly, relaxed and aware of your surroundings, until you feel ready to open your eyes, revived and ready to carry on with your day.

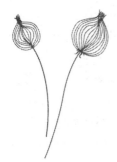

# COMING HOME
# TO YOUR BABY

*'Bright but hidden, the Self dwells in the heart.*
*Everything that moves, breathes, opens and closes*
*Lives in the Self. He is the source of love . . .'*
**The Upanishads**

You and your baby are getting to know each other face-to-face, developing lifelong bonds of love and attachment. Just being near you makes your baby feel comfortable, safe and secure within the boundaries of their small world. While you can grow to appreciate the small details of who they are: a finger wrapped around your own, the hint of a smile, their body nestling into the curve of your own, limbs stretching out in sleep.

These first few months pass by so quickly, but you already know the platitudes. This tiny human being is not going to stay like this forever. So enjoy their childhood while you can. The seeds of maternal love will continue to grow, even when you have to look up way above you to establish eye contact with your child. You will never again know the sheer delight of getting to know your baby for the first time. It's all too easy to forget that this part only happens once in a lifetime. And now is that time!

## Breaking the ice

Truly get to know your baby. This is all there really is to do. After childbirth, you redefine the physical dynamic between the two of you, outside of the protective sphere of your body. It takes time to adjust to a mother-and-child relationship, as two separate human beings. Spend quiet time with your baby each day, just being in each other's presence and nurturing the instinctive bonds between you. Without other people staking a claim over your time and attention.

You may want to resist the intensity of change. You don't always want to be a mother figure living in a new baby world. It's something you have to reconnect to each day afresh. The starting point is to appreciate, value and enjoy the time with your children, even when you're not doing much. This is the foundation upon which your relationship will grow and flourish.

## Your home is a sanctuary

Your home is not just a concrete building of bricks and mortar. It is a place in which you store your family's hopes and aspirations, where you find happiness, fulfilment and identity. You can find the reflection of who you are in the surroundings you create around you. Some days, it feels like a castle of dreams, a haven of peace; others, a prison cell or demolition site. As a mother you need to feel safe, secure and protected when you are at home. When you set foot inside the threshold, you are able to leave the rest of the world on your doorstep, unless you invite it in.

Your front door opens and you have access to a sanctuary where you are safe to revitalize and recuperate with your baby. Stepping into a mothering cocoon where you are comfortable and at ease, well as far as you can be. This space is essential, especially when going out anywhere involves a physical battle grappling with buggies or slings, changing bags and car seats. It is up to you to send away any wolves that threaten to blow down your

## BREATHING ALONGSIDE YOUR BABY

Lie down next to your baby, making sure you are both warm and comfortable. Take time to really look at this tiny human being, the extraordinary details of them: their tiny fingers, toes and nails all perfectly formed and shaped, the soft down of their hair, their bright sparkling eyes turning toward your voice, their abandonment in sleep, the snuffling, grunting noises when feeding, the exquisite softness of their skin.

Get to know who this little person is. See your baby's vitality, how they express themselves, whether waving arms or legs around, singing, grumbling or slowly drifting off to sleep. Notice how they breathe, the shallow and rapid rise and fall of their chest. Synchronize your breath with theirs, linking your breath into a pattern, even if not a mirror image of their own. Allow your breath tone to resonate with your child's, the thread of universal energy linking you together.

sense of security and stability. So you always have a haven where you can be vulnerable. Create a home where you switch off, let go and relax in a space that truly is your own.

## Drawing boundaries around family life

Your baby's arrival may herald an explosion of phone calls and visitors, all wanting to give their personal blessings and well wishes to your family. In the early days and weeks after childbirth, the whole world and its neighbouring planets want to share a slice of your family's time and attention. Yet you haven't even got to know each other yet, let alone become used to the new dynamic of living together. The intense gaze of public attention may be the last thing on earth that you want, as you arrive out of childbirth, vulnerable, battered and still on the mend. You want to enjoy your baby in tranquility, without keeping up with the demands of making cups of tea for visitors and clearing up cake crumbs afterwards, while everyone gets to hold and cuddle your baby except you.

It is natural to feel a sense of dislocation while adjusting to the differences between your life, before and after giving birth. The centripetal force of maternal love draws you toward your baby, not to the social externalities of playing hostess to other adults. You may have been warned about the invasive visitor syndrome. The conflict between needing undiluted time with your baby, without having to fit in around other adults' schedules. So drop the amnesia and remember your priorities: to restore your energy levels and concentrate on getting to know your baby, doing both on your own terms. You don't have to circle around on the periphery while your baby is obliged to make a star appearance across your social life. You are the mother in all this. It is your prerogative to decide how many visitors you want to see, while also keeping your sanity. No one else needs to assume a director's role here except you.

You owe yourself the right to recuperate and heal after childbirth. Everything else can wait. So what's the worst that is going to happen? Great

Aunty Daisy will feel bothered and mutter about being kept waiting on the doorstep. But she is not living inside your shoes. You decide where you are going to place your feet as a mother. And when you are ready to welcome other people in; and when you want them to leave. Live with sincerity, so you don't suffer from visitor intrusion, or start to resent all the contacts in your address book in the process.

Each day is a day spent or lost with your baby. Have integrity and focus on what matters to you, whatever your emotions are screaming at you. Your emotional landscape draws your mind back toward the centre point of your being: to trust your maternal feelings and instincts, and give love and nurture to your baby. And you don't need anyone else to teach or show you how to do this.

There is no reason to feel a misplaced sense of obligation or guilt when you put up a closed sign on the window, and retreat into the centre of your nuclear family. You can also choose to only see people who support you unconditionally, rather than inadvertently draining your energy levels. Your baby doesn't know or care whether they miss a social foray into another adult's arms. There is all the time in the world to make meaningful connections. That will come. The only people that your child wants to be with are you, your partner and other siblings.

## Strengthening the nucleus of your family

You have spent nine months waiting to meet your child – so don't give this over to the agendas of other people, before you even start. You can appreciate the love and kindness of others from a distance. What is most important is that that you remain happy, resilient and grounded, so you manage your mothering life as it suits you. Starting as you mean to go on. This is your absolute prerogative. Respect your autonomy, and put your family's wellbeing at the top of your concerns, rather than at the end of a draining board full of dirty dishes, as you wash your guests' empty cups and saucers.

Asserting your personal boundaries facilitates a happy and stable family relationship, rather than trying to please everyone else at the edges. You can't keep everyone happy. When your immediate family unit is thriving, then everything else falls into a natural order and place, and you can share your wellbeing with those around you.

If other people truly have your best interests at heart, they will respect and empathize with your priorities. It is better that they visit you when you have enough patience, goodwill and kindness to share with them. Say 'no' when you want to, and be the mother that you are, not the woman you think you *should* be.

## Becoming a child's guardian

We want our children to grow up to be self-aware, confident individuals, ready to stretch their wings and fly in 18 years or so. We aspire to give our young offspring the opportunities they need to grow into happy and healthy people, resilient and ready to meet life's challenges. As responsible parents, we try to have a good influence on our children's developing minds, filtering our own likes and dislikes, ideas, tastes and values, to give them a positive impression of being human.

In the early years, we decide the content of our children's lives carefully – from choice of playgroups, child-minders, pre-schools, play-dates, lifestyle, activities and diet. The years pass by, until we wake up and our eleven-year-old is telling us exactly how and where they want to get their hair cut. We have to let go of the compass of parental control sooner or later, recognizing that our child is becoming capable and mature enough to make some, if not all of their decisions.

Yet at the beginning, your child depends on you to take responsibility for the entire structure of their life. We hope to inspire and guide our offspring as they develop, so they'll be ready one day to jump into adulthood, led by their own unique life purpose – even when we don't have a clue what this is going to be. We may be tempted to assume a mantle of ownership over our

---

**TREADING LIGHTLY**

You are the temporary custodian of this human being's life. While a child might be 'yours' in the practical sense of looking after them, this little individual is never going to be a permanent possession to keep. So let go of any lasting sense of ownership, and give yourself freedom to step lightly across your child's life as their mother. Enjoying the baby that they are now, without needing a remote-control button to decide what they may become.

---

child. So we treat them like a possession. They are going to like the things we like, or do everything we weren't able to, or didn't do as a child. Until we find out that they don't want to. It's not easy to step back and let the pendulum swing away from our adult interference, to let our child be free to grow up in the direction they choose to go.

There is no guarantee that this tiny human life is going to obey or listen to your adult advice. However unbiased, valuable and well meaning you feel it is. Your role is to be a guardian, not a dictator or magician of the future. The most precious gift you have to give is unconditional love and acceptance, no strings attached. Give your child the freedom to find themselves, in shadow and light. To realize that they will be fine, even when they make mistakes. Ultimately you cannot decide who this child is going to be. Already, they are distinct, separate and complete, even while sheltering under your parental umbrella through childhood. Love them for what they bring into your life, without needing them to belong to you.

## Taming aspirations of dictatorship

Socializing your child is a vital and central part of your life as a mother. How else will they understand, feel empathy and witness the cause and effect of human behaviour in relation to themselves and others? On a more immediate level, our priorities may be to stop them from jumping on the table when we take them out to tea. To learn the basics of civility and moderation, so they are easier to live with. Most of us only have finite supplies of patience and endurance, which rapidly deplete when our offspring are running wild. In short, it is in your long-term interests to help your child to become a pleasant, considerate living companion.

Like a king's court, we may resort to persuasion, bribery or coercion to get our child to walk on the right side of what we want. We orchestrate elaborate carrot-and-stick systems: time-out, counting to three, screen time, pocket money, late nights and puddings. We then do the reverse, if the mood blows in the opposite direction. It can feel immensely difficult to get this little person to comply, as we might like, without some sort of emotional tussle. Our offspring simply don't want to be told what to do, least of all by us, and definitely not in that tone of voice. Neither do we, either now or then.

It's easy to create a schism of tension between our child and us. The ego likes to feel in control of its destiny. We want to feel acknowledged, secure and unchallenged, so a child's resistance provokes fears of anarchy and revolt against the rules of our mothering reign. Even if the assailant is only a two-year-old throwing their peas on the floor in disgust.

Children quickly discover the power of saying 'no', putting our authority on the line and placing our ethics and morality under siege. Our adult ego feels it is being attacked; suddenly there is a war to win. Although we don't mean to, we give orders to make our voice heard. We demand to be listened to and obeyed without question. Right now or else! Our relationships quickly disintegrate into an inter-generational battle of willpower, a survival-of-the-fittest contest, in which the winner appears to take control.

It's worth remembering that we are adults, not children. And can get extremely heated and prickly when trying to keep our lives vaguely on track, let alone drive them forward in the right direction. Our child may find some of our daily concerns totally irrelevant and boring. Their priorities and our own are not meant to be the same. If we weren't so engaged in the linear pursuit of our own life, we might find it easier to step back and laugh. To see the funny side of our power struggles, tiny person versus big person, even as our child winds us up like a clockwork toy. As it is, we are often too busy reacting to the emotional buttons that our child is pressing. So we fight and bite back when our authority is threatened and under fire. We desperately try to redefine our ego's place at the centre of our universe. Because if we don't do this, then what and who are we? We are so frightened that we might actually be nothing when we are exposed and vulnerable, and our personal fortifications come crashing down.

At the end of the day nobody wins. No one likes living in a domestic war zone. Yet children and adults alike still seem to constantly provoke, argue and snipe at each other in a skirmish of wills. We might secretly empathize with our child's cause. Yet we dare not risk saying so. We raise the stakes, using anger, guilt, martyrdom and dogged persistence to win a point of honour, to prove ourselves. We enforce a 'no pudding if you don't eat up' rule without mercy. Yet two florets of broccoli left on a child's plate don't really constitute a decline into chaos. So how does a difference of opinion escalate into a major battle of egos? What is all of this really about?

We all exist in a perpetual state of flux and change, yet find it so hard to accept that we are not solid and fixed in stone. Already, your baby is developing new skills and reaching milestones that are different from yesterday's. You can't hang on to who they once were, except as an idea that doesn't now exist. We never truly get used to our impermanence, clinging to a deep-rooted desire to build security, stability and permanence in life. Our ego has a survival reflex of wanting to be in control, and our children shake its boundaries. When challenged, we feel the raw points of our vulnerability. And we know that life is fragile and can easily fall apart.

So it's likely that you will always insist that vegetables are a vital part of a growing toddler's diet, and wellingtons (rubber boots) are worn when splashing through muddy puddles. There is a cut-off point when 'no' really does mean 'NO' in big capital letters! But you don't have to win all the battles, without making any exceptions to the rules. There is grace and strength in conceding defeat. In not always having to prove you are right,

**KEEPING CONFLICT UNDER CONTROL**

Breathe out deeply when your ego is spiralling out of control. Stand back and look at your child, so determined to stand their ground over a plate of peas. Remember how it feels to be small and overwhelmed by a plate of vegetables. How difficult it can be to find a way back from conflict, even as an adult. How much more so when you are a child trying to understand what is the best thing to do.

Take the initiative and diffuse conflict when you can, so there is a chance to move forward from impasse. Together. There isn't any parenting device in the world that will get your children to always agree with you. Sometimes, the change will have to come from within you. So let your child have a turn at standing their ground. Yes, your intentions may be noble and pure – to bring your children up to be chivalrous, decent members of society. Yet you won't do this by pushing or pulling them into shape, without also drawing out empathy, cooperation and respect.

even if you secretly think you are! Conserve your fighting spirit for the big issues. Choose your battles wisely, and see if you can make victory into a joint venture, so everyone has a chance of winning.

## Moving beyond your control reflex

Do you constantly tell your child what to do; also how and when to do it as well? If you suspect so, you give your offspring little choice but to fight back, give up or else retreat from you. Either way, you are motivating them into a state of mutiny. And they will probably still find a way to disagree with you, even when you insist otherwise. You don't want to provoke anger, insecurity or silent resentment. What happens when you release your hold over your family's control panel? Try stepping back to let your partner and children move forward to enjoy shared ownership over your mutual lives together. When you move away from the frontline of domestic strife, you can coexist peacefully, engaging with those you love without conflict.

The challenge is to find a harmonious living dynamic with other people, without needing to prove our validity. Does it matter whether we are right, better or stronger than anyone else. Recognize when it does. We so often say 'no' as a reflex, when what we really mean is, 'I don't like that, but only because I am different from you.' There doesn't need to be a judgment, only acknowledgement and acceptance of difference.

You will never be able to truly jump into your child's mind or see the world through their eyes. You can only listen acutely, and try to empathize with their point of view. And this will bring you to understanding them. So then you can offer and give your child some realistic choices, so they are able to learn how to cooperate, bend *and* make their own decisions. Without always being forced to agree with you or pushed into defiance. Peas or carrots is a simple enough choice, yet empowers a child to know what they want, and to take responsible action to achieve this. This gives them a solid foundation of self-confidence, high self-esteem and an understanding of how to create a positive train of cause and effect in their lives.

Do you actually believe you know everything that is going to happen today or tomorrow? Of course not! So where did we get this notion that the rich and varied pattern of the universe is subject to the rule of our individual ego. The most we can do is understand ourselves, and the impact we create around us. Before we even start to take account of the myriad of other possibilities that might also come to pass. The only thing we can decide is how and where we place our feet with each step we take, leaving a happy trail of footprints behind us.

## Non-attachment

We are spontaneously affectionate to the people and objects we like. We love someone because it feels good. So we want more of this. We're soon addicted to these feel-good emotions, looking to those we love to fulfil our fragile sense of wellbeing. Our love, once freely given, becomes entangled in strings of attachment; we need other people to fulfil this craving within us. On the other hand, we can't wait to push away our dislikes and hates, especially when they come too close to us. We push away those parts of people's characters that provoke strong feelings of aversion. It is hard work to find equanimity when your emotions are telling you a different story.

To love your child deeply and passionately is a natural part of the bonding process. Yet, it doesn't follow that you automatically relish all the practicalities of looking after them, just because you adore them. Who really enjoys waking up in the middle of the night to feed and settle a restless baby, month after month? So there will be aspects that just don't do it for you: battling with bottles, leaky nappies (diapers), buggies and car seats, while also managing heavy bags of shopping isn't much fun. It's easy to fall into a trap of only welcoming the nice, pleasant bits of mothering, while trying to shove away the rest of it. This doesn't work in practice. Yes, there are things that we like or else hate, depending on the stimuli. And we react accordingly, craving more or less of the same. Yet, you're still stuck with the less salubrious bits of daily childcare, but may be so busy resenting them, that you're less able to deal constructively with them.

The deep wellspring of maternal love quickly gets clogged up when we cling on to feelings of attachment or aversion. We don't always decide our feelings. Yet we can choose how we relate these back to the specific high and low points of our daily childcare routine. We are slaves to our emotions. We place great emotional value on the good and happy times, easy enough to do when things are smooth and flowing. Yet we become fraught with disappointment and suffering when we don't find this place. You are a part of the universe, and the universe exists within you. And love is present within you, regardless of your feelings, no strings attached.

## Concentrating on what really is important

As a mother, we want to be able to hold our attention steady, quiet and unwavering when family storms are brewing. To draw our energy away from the external maelstrom, and keep our inner gaze fixed firmly on our heart centre. This is the practice of *Pratyahara*. When we retrain our mind to respond with calm awareness, rather than raw emotion to the family dramas that our senses generate about us. We don't add more fuel to the tempest stewing in the domestic teacup. Instead, we focus on remaining alert, poised and at ease, when emotional whirlwinds blow up, as they will from time to time in your family's life.

When you practise withdrawing your senses from the scene of emotion, you are able to respond with equanimity to the forming crisis. You can channel your energy into riding this wave of sensation, without falling head first into it. This is more than we could possibly hope for in any average day!

We all know that the cocktail of mixing our children's moods with our own can be highly unpredictable, volatile and often directly influenced by our surroundings. So when you come head-to-head with a widening fault line, learn to hold yourself steady. At least sometimes! Keep your emotions in focus through discomforting circumstances. So you literally raise your mind, lifting it up and beyond the reach of storm clouds. And from this point of clarity, you can see the great expanse of consciousness stretching out away from the dramas.

### PRACTICING INNER FOCUS

Take a common mothering scenario. Your baby has woken up grouchy and won't stop grizzling and grumbling. You've tried feeding, burping, rocking, singing and dancing to distract them into a good mood for the last hour or so. Yet it's not working. And your patience is wearing thin. Your emotions are starting to rise, as your baby's decibels increase. The ambience is slowly shifting. You can feel the first signs of frustration stirring, as your senses start pulling you into the hurricane zone of mother-and-baby discontent.

The one thing you can always do is keep your attention centred on your breath. Don't let go of your concentration, stop breathing or hyperventilate under the pressure! Keep your concentration steady, focused on finding space within the breath, unchanging, constant in the face of the rising storm. Remain present without spiralling off at a tangent. Slowly your senses will stop pulling your emotions like elastic, as you plant and ground your energy into a state of inner peace and stillness. Be present to the drama and let it pass over you, so you can direct a finale that you want.

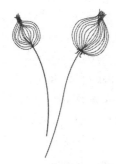

# BUILDING MOTHERING BRIDGES

*'We live in this world when we love it.'*
**Rabindranath Tagore**

If you are always too busy being an adult, you cannot get to know your child. How can you find out who this child actually is, if you are already rushing past them? When you slow down your living pace, you can empathize and understand your child's perspective, seeing their unique priorities and feelings as they are.

We tend to forget what it is like to be a child, even though we were once young ourselves. When you listen to and engage with your child's viewpoint, it can unlock a storehouse of memories of childhood, locked away since you grew up. Your own legacy of childhood can guide you as a parent, enriching your child's life now, as they grow up in the present. You can do things differently, filling your child's path with happiness and delight. Your personal empathy with the child you once were is a profound tool to help you to understand and relate to what your child is feeling, saying and talking about now.

So, as a mother, open your heart to perceive the world through your child's eyes. Stepping away from the fortress of your adult concerns, you can rediscover simple pleasures, discovering life afresh again each day. Enjoy the experience of switching off your phone, and taking a whole afternoon to walk a short distance and back again with your child. You won't need anything else other than each other and what you can see around you to find joy through what you create inside your heart. Take time to stop, transfixed by the floating pattern of a falling leaf, daylight fading, raindrops hanging from leaves, early morning mists rising, the call of a songbird or a rain-soaked road steaming in sunshine. The art of simplicity transforms each moment into a playground for you and your children.

## Opening your perspective

Put down the mask of adult self-consciousness and discover experiences you have missed or forgotten. Walk barefoot on dew-soaked grass, feel rain on your face without flinching, feel the warmth of sunshine on your skin, feel the wind against your back with arms wide open, splash in puddles wearing wellingtons (rubber boots), make a daisy chain, find animals in the clouds, walk over the cracks in pavements, notice the beauty in the world as it is. And tell stories to your child about your adventures together. Dissolve any complacency that you've seen and done it all before. Clear your perspective without depending on your past interpretation of how things are. You can only ever know how life is now: fresh, and each moment a new beginning.

## Empathy and listening

When our children speak to us, we often answer them before they even finish the sentence. How can you be so sure you know what they are going to say? You don't need to, and can't discern what they want to communicate, before they articulate their feelings themselves. You aren't supposed to have supernatural powers; a super-mama who is aware of everything, about anything, before your child even says a word. When you don't listen and actually hear what your child wants to share with you, you are missing a gateway into their personal world. Failing to catch hold of the trust they are reaching out to give you.

It is not your remit as a parent to know it all, before your child's life has begun. Even if we might have a fair idea of what they are likely to say or do in the short term, before they may know this for themselves. We often spend much of our life following a script that we don't consciously seem to be writing. So we don't always reach a happy conclusion. We tend to know how we're going to act and behave, before we do. We can predict our reactions, because we don't bother to stop and engage our hearts in what we're thinking, doing or communicating. We ignore the infinite possibilities outside of our immediate blueprint of obvious responses. Intent on following a well-trodden path of dialogue, even if this doesn't really resolve any of the questions asked. It's hardly surprising that we rarely delight or amaze ourselves in our answers or actions.

How often do you truly stop and listen to what your child is saying to you? If you are busy talking or doing something else, you may miss what they are trying to express. Sure, we can easily give a direct explanation to a three-year-old looking for clarity on how electricity works. Yet at some point, it helps to find silence. To stop the train of mental rationalizing, justifying, analyzing, explaining and churning-out of words.

As the flow of dialogue calms down, our stream of consciousness quietens, and we develop sensitivity and intuition, to sense what is really being said underneath the surface. How often do we say one thing, mean another and then do something totally different? In listening with clarity and insight, we learn to tread gently through our relationships, without trampling on the sentiment given within the choice of language. We understand what is not

RECOGNIZING YOUR VOICE TONE

Listen to the timbre and feeling tone of your voice. What can you hear beyond the literal meaning of your words? We often prefer to remain ignorant, oblivious to the true sentiment of emotion running through our dialogue. But this message is ringing out as clear as a bell. It can be so much easier and convenient to ignore our true intention, to shut our ears to what we are really saying. To speak without feeling. Yes, our words might sound impressive, proving to all and sundry that we know what we are talking about. Yet it is the heart's wisdom that creates truth and meaning, not the narrative that we often dwell on needlessly. This wisdom gives our words true significance.

So catch yourself before you start a stream of talking. Take a couple of breaths before your thoughts solidify into a trail of words behind you. If you don't like what you hear, how do you think your family find it! So spend a day listening, rather than talking, and see what you learn about yourself and others around you. What do your family reveal in their use of words and body language? Do you speak out of choice, desire or force of habit?

To communicate is to truly acknowledge and accept the presence of someone else, as they truly are. We all want to give and receive the gift of undivided attention to those we love, to show that we care. Are you able to be receptive to your children or is your mind already moving on to other things? Open up a channel between your voice and heart, building a bridge with the words you use.

being said, as well as what we hear around us. We can see beyond the words that are offered to us.

## Creating the sound of happiness

You paint a verbal picture with your words. Observe what you are creating in the choice of language you use. You have the power to fill a blank canvas with language. So be careful what you leave behind, as each day passes. What motivates you to speak, and do you really want your children to carry this around with them? Deep down, you already know when you are speaking to hurt, judge, put down or criticize. When you spin words to weave a self-image to deceive everyone, including yourself. Too often we speak to prove ourselves, filling in the gaps, to make us feel whole inside.

We may find we use our words as a weapon to destroy those who appear as a threat or obstacle in our way. Suddenly we are in a dialogue of harsh explosives and emotional tirades. We say so much more than we mean to, and then come to regret this later, wishing we could take it back again. Clear the slate. Listen to the ambience of your words left hanging in the space around you. What is the nature of the emotional residue that you are leaving behind, long after the physical vibration of your voice has faded away?

You may have a radically different point of view from your partner or children. Can your find a way around this, to affirm and show you care about them? To create communication of lasting value out of the positive sentiment of the words you use. You can build self-confidence, esteem and security in your children, even when you disagree with their interpretation of how the mechanics of family life work. They have one opinion and you have another. So stop and listen, and then communicate from the undercurrent of love that runs between you and your children.

## Finding silence

When your mind and body are peaceful, there is silence. Let your words arise from a wellspring of boundless stillness, falling back again into its depths.

When you are motivated by your inner wisdom, your words are shaped with truth, rather than jumping out of an impetuous mind. You already know when you are speaking for the greater good, motivated by a pure intention that encourages kindness, consideration and generosity of speech. There is nothing to gain when you don't communicate using this motivation. There is already so much suffering in the world, so much harshness, cruelty, hurt and tears. You don't really want to add more to this stockpile of misery, especially in your own home.

So think carefully about what your intention is and how you can express this, before you bring it out into the open. The silence, the meaning of what you are saying, can speak more poignantly than a million words. Use stillness to find momentum to express your own vulnerability and humanity, giving love to those around you.

## Building bridges of connection

Connect with your baby by gently weaving a carpet of nurture under them with your voice, touch and eyes. There is always time to be aware of, and show how much you adore and cherish this little person, whenever you make contact with them: when you reach down to change them, blow raspberries on their tummy, comfort them with a cuddle, rub their back after a feed. Giving your child a constant supply of love and nurture through your presence, you can consciously raise the vibration of your interactions with them, so you are genuinely expressing love.

Channeling your intuition through your senses, you cultivate and deepen the bonds of love, trust and nurture that exist between you and your baby. In bridging the gap between your different realities, you re-experience the intimacy of pregnancy and reaffirm bonds of connection. This enhances your baby's emotional capacity to recognize and cherish loving relationships, to relate to the world outside.

Your baby instinctively turns toward the comfort of being near you. They seek you out, trusting that they will always find you. Holding your essence, your sound, smell and aura within their mind, heart and body. Each time you reach out and make contact with your baby, you reinforce firm foundations of knowing themselves through you.

## Baby massage

Your baby instinctively turns to you, needing to be held in your arms. You can use touch to stimulate your baby's development and wellbeing by using gentle massage from birth. Your hands are wonderful tools to connect with your young baby, helping them to feel safe and secure in their world. Showing your child that you care about them, sharing love and appreciation for their small life. This helps your baby to make sense of their separate existence, to adjust to the immensity of being divided from your pregnant body. As you massage your child, you reignite your deep connection to them. This helps you to tune into the non-verbal cues that your baby is constantly giving you, about how things are in their small world.

You do not need expert guidance on how to do baby massage. The most important thing is that you both enjoy this experience. Your baby massage time will soon be an occasion that you both look forward to, where you can feel relaxed, happy and enjoy being together. As well as being a pleasure, gentle massage is incredibly beneficial to your baby's development and growth. Releasing feel-good endorphins, it aids optimum functioning of the digestive, circulatory and respiratory systems. It also provides sensory and muscular stimulation for your baby's mind and body and promoting spatial awareness. Research also suggests that gentle massage can alleviate colic, releasing trapped wind in the digestive system and help your baby to settle and sleep.

You need enough time to enjoy the process of giving a massage, without rushing through it from start to finish. Give your baby a massage when they are less likely to be hungry or fussy; it can take anything between 5 and 30 minutes. It may make them feel very sleepy, so be ready to stop if they start napping before you have finished. Some days, it will be a longer session, other times a few minutes is enough. Just go with whatever feels right. Relax and let go of any physical tension before you start: shrugging your shoulders, stretching your arms out and taking a few deep breaths to arrive home in your body.

Give your whole attention to your baby: engage your sense of touch, and connect to a deeper consciousness flowing inside your own mind and body. You may feel that you often have little time to stop and be truly present to your baby. There is always so much to do; one nappy (diaper) change and feeding time blends into the next. So massage is a wonderful space to be with your young baby, with no motivation other than to spend undiluted time in each other's company. Here, you can stop, rest and catch your breath before you pick up the rest of your daily chores and routine.

## BABY MASSAGE TECHNIQUE

You need a warm, cozy room so your baby is comfortable. Take off their clothes, covering them with a blanket. (Leave their nappy/diaper on, unless you're happy to clean up any accidents!) Because your baby is so small, they cannot regulate their body temperature as effectively as you can, so minimize draughts and turn the heating up, so the room is warm enough. Your baby can lie on their back on a rug, with a towel beneath them to prevent any mess. Adjust the lighting to a soft glow, and put on soothing music if this helps you both to relax.

Ask for your baby's permission to give them a massage. Even if they can't actually reply back to you, this respects your child's personal space when they can't articulate a response about their preferences. Use baby massage oil or sweet almond base oil. The basic technique is to use a very gentle and non-intrusive touch, remaining receptive to how your baby responds. As your baby's body is very fragile, use a gentle, soft pressure, only as much as a fingertip pressed down comfortably on a closed eyelid. Nothing more.

You will develop your own massage routine, working from the right to the left side of the body. Be aware of your baby's anatomy, the hard bony structures and soft tissues. You could try stroking up along the body, gently squeezing out arms and legs, making tiny circles with a finger, smoothing out the skin. Listen to what your baby and your own hands are telling you, and discover what feels right and comfortable for you both. You can gently move your baby's arms and legs to encourage the limbs to move and open, working within the natural limitations of your baby's movements. After a few minutes, you will start to sense, or else your baby will tell you, that it's time to stop. So draw things to a close. Try to time your session so you end on a good note.

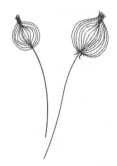

# MATERNAL LOVE

*'The earth is your mother,*
*she holds you.*
*The sky is your father,*
*he protects you.*
*We are together, always.*
*We are together, always.*
*There was never a time*
*when this was not so.'*
**Navajo lullaby**

We spend most of our lives searching for a source of love, unconditional, constant and whole. As a foetus, we found this union living within the safety and security of our mother's womb. There was no separation between our two lives. And then came the moment of birth, and an immense sense of dislocation. In taking our first independent breath, we connect to our destiny to be separate and alone. We become an individual; someone who is distinct and unique from all other living forms in the universe. And yet who is also the same. And now your baby has made the same journey.

We understand the world around us through our senses. The brain interprets our sensory cues, then makes sense of the world around us as something that is different and set apart from us. Since the time spent in our mother's womb, we experience a sense of spiritual disconnection, cut off from the living source of our energy that brought us into human existence.

The experience of being an integral part of the universe fades into insignificance, until we no longer remember or know it anymore. We have forgotten that our life started in harmony, existing as part of our mother's womb. Instead, we start to define the rest of humanity in terms of 'here's me, and there's you'. We put away our natural sense of interconnectedness with the planet, displacing our natural ability to live in synergy with our surroundings. Even when we do live and express our humanity with passion, creativity and integrity, we still do so as an individual. We can spend an entire lifetime searching to reconnect with a living sense of union with the universe. To find a higher source of divinity that remains buried deep within us.

As a young baby, you re-experience union, completeness, while breast-feeding, or lying in the warm embrace of your mother's arms. However, children are quickly taught to grow up and stand firmly on their own two feet. Our social conditioning makes us value ourselves as an individual first and foremost. Our nuclear family becomes our immediate priority, the global one less so. The reality is that we are one part of a universal family of humanity, living on a shared planet of resources. Yet this is often little more than a cognitive idea, that doesn't really impact on us. We stop short of integrating the truth of our wholeness back into our heart, to make it part of our emotional framework of living.

So while we might accept we are all part of the same oneness in theory, we don't let ourselves recognize this in living practice. We stop short of allowing our heart to merge with the universe, heal wounds, let down our guard and find togetherness with the rest of the human species. We think that the only way to get on in life – whether that is in the playground, school or career – is to defend our fragile individuality from the dangerous world outside. We wrap up our true feelings inside a protective cloak of personality, hiding away our vulnerability. We try to prove that we are complete, intact and doing fine. We fear exposure: that it will be discovered that we aren't any stronger, better or worse than anybody else.

Why do we still find it so hard to be satisfied with our human lot, except in short-lived bursts of self-gratification and indulgence? Even with all the sensory pleasures in the galaxy and beyond. The big wide world stretches out around us. It is never enough, because we don't look within ourselves. When we let our guard down, it turns out that we have the same hopes, fears and dreams as each and every other human being on the planet. We think we are not enough, because we are unable to see what we already are.

We can find the way back home within ourselves. To the divine source of benevolence running through us, that leads us to manifest peace, joy and contentment in our life. In learning to be us, yet finding an authentic connection with everybody else as well, the heart awakens to rejoice in the simple truth that we are not alone.

## Learning to love

Many of us forget how to give and receive love and compassion freely, without attaching rules and preconditions. Sure, we feel happy and loving sometimes, if not all of the time. Yet we still depend on something else, anything except ourselves, to enable us to experience happiness, satisfaction and contentment. We need people, places and the things around us, to feel good about being alive. As long as we imprison our hearts within these trappings, we continue to suffer disappointment, rejection, hurt and pain.

We tend to act like a performing monkey, thinking we will only find love if we behave like this or that. Love becomes a commodity in our life with prerequisites attached. We develop maxims – 'I love you when you are like this, but I'm not sure I do when you do that.' The clarity and boundless nature of love becomes fragmented by our needs and desires. It trickles down to form a meagre portion of our relationships. The awakened, expansive nature of the heart lies dormant.

We all have sublime experiences, when we love without boundaries and inhibition. When we step into the light of pure awareness, touching our divinity, consciousness, goodness, we interconnect with all living things. We may feel an exquisite tenderness for our children, partners, family and friends; the sweetness of love and affection links us like a bridge, connecting our hearts together. Our hearts can be awakened by another's suffering, and we drop into a river of pure compassion that encompasses everyone around us without exception. A stranger's life touches us and we feel their happiness or pain as our own.

## Completing the circle

In fleeting moments of purity, something immense and beautiful happens. A fellow human being's existence opens a river of love and compassion in our heart. We start to soften, thaw and let go; feeling vulnerable, exposed, yet vibrantly alive. The heart cracks open, and suddenly we are overflowing with empathy, joy and wellbeing. The defensive fortress of ego, which creates such barricades between the universe and us, is washed away.

As the heart awakens to bliss, it expands to encompass the limitless expanse of humanity, stretched out across the planet's surface. You experience a profound and exquisite sense of union, completeness and belonging, as the boundaries of your personal identity dissolve into your true universal nature. And then, as with all things, life changes again, the moment passes, and you are back living within the divisive illusion of self and other. There's me, and everything else that isn't a part of me. Once again, we're playing out our patterns of thoughts and emotions, from force of habit. Until the next moment of clarity comes to greet us.

Joy and spontaneity have the capacity to transform your perception of life. Cleansing your perspective, you are able to see things differently, not just in the moment, but when it passes. A fleeting sense of infinite love and compassion make a clear imprint on your mind of your heart's true nature, forming a lasting impression. You may try to recapture this sublime feeling of union and wholeness within you, wanting no other substitute than this. We then search to find our way back through the labyrinth of mind to this inner source of living grace. This becomes our true life's purpose. To uncover the heart's living presence inside us and embrace this gift of universal love, divinity, God, the absolute, reality and goodness. This is enough.

## The push and pull of nurture

You can only stop being a mother in the early months, when you hand over the mantle of your baby's care to someone else for a short while. Unless you are lucky, you may not have this get-out clause readily available to use when you need it. Your supply of willing grandparents, family and friends with a free pair of hands, may not meet your demand for them. So the constant responsibility of looking after your baby may quickly erode your sense of autonomy and freedom. You have to put so many other things on hold and spring into action whenever your child needs you. This displacement of self may feel like your energy is being pulled out of your body and fed into a black hole. In truth, having a baby can make you feel very old, tired and weary – like a puppet working non-stop on its worn-out strings.

These are tricky times. When you just can't seem to get your baby to stop crying, grizzling, whinging or shouting. They absolutely insist that their rightful place to be is in your arms, refusing to leave you without protesting for even one short second. Creating an instant commotion in a thousand and one ways when they want attention that you either don't have or want to give just now. The centripetal force of your baby's presence, gives you no other choice but to follow them, albeit reluctantly, to the centre of their universe. For no reason than you are their mother, and on duty. You become your own worst enemy if you try to fight the intense pull of maternal nurture.

So moments may arise when you know you love your baby, but oh dear, you're not sure that you have the strength to believe this with any conviction. On the contrary, you're stewing an emotional broth of lethargy, frustration, despair, anger, irritation, impatience and guilt. Like an internal pressure cooker coming up to the boil with a faulty release valve, you blow. Sometimes you long for a few minutes without having to deal with your baby, who is reminding you with awesome persistence that this isn't possible. At least not for another few more years! While love may be unconditional, your capacity to nurture may have a decidedly finite nature!

This is not an issue about caring, because you do. You love your baby madly, passionately and deeply with every cell in your body. But you still have days when you temporarily misplace your maternal instincts, and can do nothing to smooth away the rough surfaces of full-time parenting. You are staggering under the emotional burden of having to placate your child for the umpteenth time. And even though you know that it needs to be done, so it will be done, this realization doesn't help your feelings. If anything, it makes you even more emotional and weepy.

'Where is the love?' you might ask yourself quietly, so as not to hurt the baby's feelings. 'And why can't I find any joy, peace or fulfilment when I need them?' This is where your mothering journey of inner growth truly begins, in the moments when your maternal inspiration is in short supply or spent. And you are suffering from a drought of caring. All you actually want is to put your head in the sand, or preferably just lie down. Instead you're suffocating in tedious monotony, dragging your emotional heaviness around, through yet another solitary afternoon spent with a young baby.

The crux of the matter is that you 'have to' be a parent, because there is no other option available. There isn't a manufacturer's guarantee that comes with childbirth, which enables you to recharge your love for your baby. And while every other job you've done had some sort of annual leave allowance, you're literally in a parenting job for life. Even if you have obliging grandparents to lean on, or the financial means and inclination to buy in respite, you still have to face motherhood at times when you don't want to. And keep trying to give your best to your children every day of your life.

Ultimately you know that you're still the best candidate for the role of being the mother of your children. This job is meant for you alone. When you are at your lowest point, remember that deep down under the pile of dirty nappies (diapers) building up, there really is a source of pure radiant love inside you. And if those nappies decided to bounce up and down on your sleeping baby, well you would fight them with your last breath to protect this little person's life that you love so much. Let your spirit rise back up to the surface, cleansing and bathing you and your baby in wellbeing. Helping you find enough to get by on.

### Finding the love in the dirty laundry

Oh dear, it didn't work! You've still had enough. You're so tired, worn out, and suffering from baby fatigue. You know that you're meant to feel soft, fluffy mothering emotions, as you dole out endless supplies of patience, kindness and positive attention to your children. But the inner storehouse of 'goodness' in you is empty. There is nothing left to give. It takes real guts, integrity and determination to keep on going when you've lost faith. When you would rather give up and die for a short while. Try pretending that you're interested and engaged. Do anything but sink further down.

Take one small step forward, then another if you can manage it. Shuffle across your threshold of endurance and resilience, building up strength and resolve again, regardless of your feelings. This is about your spiritual awakening, increasing your capacity to fill up your reserves, when you are scratching against bare earth. Things will change. And when this mood passes, you will know you have found the courage to be a spiritual warrior to your children. Even when you've partially collapsed as a mother in the process!

You may still struggle to hit the mark, to find mothering love in the rising decibels of your child's shouting crescendo. When you lose sight of your emotional centre of gravity, come back into the heart. Breathe out and feel light and wellbeing at your core, a deep current flowing beneath the maternal debris. Cultivate concentration and the resolve to turn away from real or imaginary critics who judge, blame and put down your mothering capabilities. Allow yourself to be receptive to anything, except discord. If you aren't prepared to move toward the heart's light shining within you, how can you find solace in your life? Especially when things are as ghastly as they sometimes seem to be.

Your mothering resistance brings you face-to-face with one of the greatest hurdles that you will ever need to jump over in life. You need to surrender to life without trying to make it different. Let your heart open so you truly accept and connect with the human being you are. Just let things be, and grow inside, without trying to fix them with the force of willpower alone. Accept life as it is, without rejecting or fighting what you see. And keep forgiving your own shortfalls when you dissolve into anger, tears and frustration. Allow yourself to be a mother: to be exhausted, tense, downtrodden, barely hanging on, and still believe that this latest trauma can dissolve into love, patience and compassion. And then your heart will return full circle, giving hope back to you and your child.

There is no other way to arrive home! You learn to accept reality as it is, to survive this pain barrier, when your baby is inadvertently dragging you through it. You have to keep going, if only by miming the motions. Sometimes merely surviving, yet still believing in your capacity to find infinite joy and happiness. You are a mother for the rest of your life, through all of your child's journey growing up by your side. For better and worse – through the good days, the mediocre days and the plain awful days!

Keep positive, sane and self-reliant. Adjusting your mothering apron, so it expands out to fit around your personal boundaries of self and embraces your baby's presence. In surrendering, you dissolve the fight and struggle inside your mind, and arrive out into the light of acceptance.

## Connecting to your heart space

When you are centred in your heart, you become at one with the universal source of love flowing through you. Here, you can create a mothering practice, giving and receiving love and compassion without expectations, especially when things aren't going so well with your baby, partner or whoever else. Your heart opens to accept things how they are, regardless of your individual desires.

You may not want to practise love and peace when you are suffering. It may be the last thing that comes to mind when your equanimity is sliding off at a wild tangent, and things are going wrong. This quality of boundless love, wellbeing and appreciation is something that you have to cultivate; engaging with your spirit isn't always automatic. Once a living practice, you are then able to follow the scent of loving compassion back to your heart.

In being mindful of the heart, you renew the incredible relationship you create each day with your child. When your baby starts crying just after you've put your nice hot lunch on the table, be realistic about your expectations of how you will react to them. Don't try to be a saint, pretending you're not bothered when you obviously are. Acknowledge quick flashes of murky feelings, and then rest into your heart's essence. Your heart is waiting to spring into life, revitalizing you when you are crumbling. Here your emotions don't have the same power to provoke and pull you into anger and stress. They don't matter so much in your heart space. Your divine nature can stretch out, unbounded by the mutterings of your ego.

Your personal mothering challenges may bring a symphony of negative thoughts and painful emotions into chorus. You tend to fall flat on your face when you're up against the phenomena of sleepless nights, crying and fussiness. So come back to your heart's energy, recognizing love within you. How can you give love to a child, when you have so little to give back to yourself? Throw away unkind and critical thoughts, and put your attention elsewhere, so love can grow. Just one tiny drop of love is enough. Your heart starts to unfurl, opening and expanding into something more powerful, universal and greater than the individual ego's clamours for self-justification.

Offer yourself the gift of love, generosity and forgiveness, as much as you give these to your baby. You need to experience love so badly when reality doesn't follow your perfect mental blueprint, and you're suffering the consequences. The shadowy traits of personality – anger, discord, jealously, comparison, despair and bitterness – rise up, removing you from wholeness into tension. The gift of love and compassion softens your pain, without wanting or taking anything in return. No silent demands to become stoical, happier, kinder and more patient. Just loving kindness, where you thought there was none.

To find love and compassion is a blessing. Transforming each day into something unique and beautiful, to counteract the 'if onlys' and 'what ifs' holding the mind in the throes of yesterday and tomorrow. You accept you cannot necessarily change the present into something else. The mind settles into a natural state of serenity, calmness and contentment.

You may feel like a charlatan, making a grand facade in acting out loving emotions. Does it matter that you carry rage, despair, anguish and bitterness inside you? That nothing seems to resemble genuine love. Flip the coin over to the other side. Tend to other branches of new growth. There is always a more peaceful path for you to tread, leading you around the imperfections springing up around you. There is no need to fight, react or try to change things and make them better. Although situations may hurt and get under your skin, you can connect through your heart to the universe.

## Being gentle instead of lashing out

There are many ways in which we try to damage ourselves – through the harsh and negative impact of our thoughts, words and actions toward both self and others. We harden our minds to reject ourselves. We clinch our jaw with tension when we are late, we are breathless as we race through the morning, and we strain our bodies as we overburden ourselves with things to do. We may subtly punish ourselves in the emotional tone of our thoughts, using criticism, chastisement, judgment and negativity to mentally kick ourselves. We put ourselves down, even as we are hurting inside.

At the centre of our heart is love and kindness. *Ahimsa* is the notion of avoiding harm and being gentle to all living beings, including ourselves. It requires courage to take the plunge into life's uncertainty, not knowing if your decisions will end in success or failure. To love yourself is to accept where life takes you. Even when things go wrong or turn out differently. This is part of the fun of living. It may be that all you and baby manage to do today is watch the entire DVD box set of *Bob the Builder*. Enjoy it then, because this is what you're doing! Of course, you're going to question your motives if certain things become a daily occurrence. In the meantime, stop believing you're a 'bad person' whose childcare mantra is one of decadent indulgence.

So whatever you are up to, find softness at the edges, something to laugh and smile about. Some days will be easy, while in others you will need to create a bit of slack and let go of your exacting standards. You don't have to apologize, feel guilty and hastily explain why you might not be at your mothering best. Your intentions are pure. So, you needn't think anything such as 'you should', 'really must', or 'have to' about whatever you are able to do.

You only have this life to live, and just one chance to enjoy and treasure today before it passes. Appreciate whatever this turns out to be, rather than beating yourself up because of what it isn't. You don't really want to mutate into the imaginary replica of perfection that you carry around with you in

**BREATHING THE HEART OPEN**

Sitting or lying down in a comfortable position, close your eyes. Rubbing your palms together to generate warmth, place them one on top of the other on your chest, over the heart space. Breathe slowly and deeply as your breath becomes soft, relaxed and free. Let your breath settle into a natural rhythm, your body breathing itself, without trying to do this. Draw your attention to your hands' contact upon your chest, and let your breath flow into your heart space. Become aware of any sensations of warmth, heat, energy, light and expansion. Rest in quiet attention.

After you inhale, your breath naturally pauses before you exhale. Focus your inner gaze on this moment of suspension in the breath flow, resting in your heart as you do so. Only retain the inhalation within your body for a couple of moments, as long as you are comfortable with. Do not change the relaxed, rich quality of your breath tone. Exhale when your body is ready, emptying the breath from the body. After each inhalation, gently encourage your body to pause before you exhale. Observe this moment with your heart's awareness, where breath is hanging between the new and old. Your capacity to retain the breath will gradually lengthen over time. Practise for 5 to 20 cycles of breath. Then let go of any conscious sense of doing, as the breath settles into a natural rhythm again.

**FINDING THE HEART**

Breathing into your heart space, the mind is drawn into equilibrium. Observe any counter-impulse to indulge troll-like feelings of imperfection and worthlessness. You already know that you are unique, incredible and complete. Allow your suffering to dissolve in the living, breathing flow of love, pouring out from your heart. It is not worth hanging onto knots of angst, pain and fear that you trip over before you remember to forgive yourself for being you. You are alive, free and light. Let your heart dance with the sheer joy of being. Here is happiness, something that is present, as your heart becomes receptive to the world around you.

Uncover new depths of loving resolve to give to your children. The heart's breath raises the vibration of your intentions, raising your energy, inner strength and spirit. This is the resonance of love rising up within your heart space.

your head. It wouldn't be nearly as exciting and inspiring as getting to know and like who you actually are.

Consciously move away from your inner critic's condemnation. Choose to focus on anything, great or small, that lifts your spirits and affirms your intentions. This is self-acceptance: to live with grace without fighting or needing to become something else. The change happens when you are able to relax into each moment, and see what happens next as it does.

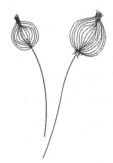

# STARTING WITH YOU

*'Be islands unto yourself, refuges unto yourselves,*
*seeking no other refuge ...'*
**Gautama Buddha,** *Mahaparinibbana Sutta*

There is nothing quite like the arrival of a newborn baby to shake up the dynamics of your relationships with family and friends. The birth of a child redefines the shape of your life, possibly more than any other life event; your own birth and death aside! It is almost as if you need to get to know the main protagonists in your life all over again afterwards, to integrate them into this new paradigm of motherhood.

You probably didn't cast a second thought about how your relationships, close and distant, might change once you've got a baby in tow. After childbirth, you're constantly arranging new maternal priorities into your life equation. Your primary concern is to be a mother first and foremost. Yet this doesn't always easily fit with what other people expect from you. After giving the best of yourself to your child all day and night, you may not have much surplus energy left to spread out at the fringes. In an ideal world, everyone would readily recognize this and empathize with a new mother's syndrome of emotional fatigue. Unfortunately in practice, you may feel you have to go way out over the halfway line to stay in contact with certain people. Even though you have little inclination or ability at the moment to do so.

It is hardly surprising that your old relationships can develop fault lines. It takes time and sensitivity for everyone to get used to you and baby being together on your own terms. You need to believe in your self-autonomy when you interact with friends and family in the outside world. So your baby's voice doesn't get drowned out by other people's calls for attention.

## Being a happy woman and a contented mother

What do you need to receive to be contented and fulfilled in your life as it now is? Listen carefully to inner cues about how you are really doing in the maternal fast lane, then honour and respect what you find out enough to act on it. Don't put off looking after your own wellbeing until later on, when the children are in bed. To consciously care for yourself is integral to being able to do the same for your children.

To manifest your own wellbeing isn't an abstract concept that you place second, behind the whirlwind of getting caught up in your children's upbringing. You need to be at your best – not only to have a fair chance of enjoying your own life, but also to find something worthwhile to share each day with your children. The common denominator of mothering fulfilment is to be receptive to what life is offering you, without wishing it were more or less. This is contentment. To be complete and grounded as a human being, so you can thrive as a woman and a mother, both with your family, and away from them. Sculpt a living canvas that reflects your love, joy and satisfaction, so both you *and* your children's spirits grow and flourish against this backdrop.

## A mother's walk forward

Find a steady mothering pace that you can sustain. You don't want to crash and burn out by the time your child can walk. You may initially pull out all the stops and levers you can to celebrate and mark the big occasions in your child's life. Yet, you're setting up an unrealistic precedence. Don't let your

---

THE RACE OF THE TORTOISE AND THE HARE

Once upon a time, a tortoise and a hare decided to have a race to see who could run the fastest. The hare was very confident that he would win by leagues, with very little effort. So the two animals set off from the starting line, the hare racing ahead into the distance, while the tortoise slowly took one small step forward at a time. After a while, the hare couldn't see the tortoise behind him. So he sat down to rest for a while. He was a very tired hare after running so fast, so he quickly fell fast asleep. In the meantime, the tortoise carried on plodding along until he passed the sleeping hare and was nearly at the finishing line. Suddenly, the hare woke up. Jumping up, he saw the tortoise in front of him in the distance, and he raced off at full speed to catch him up. It was too late. He couldn't close the gap. The tortoise slowly crossed over the finishing line winning the race, and the hare never again boasted about how fast he could run.

---

mothering quest for superlatives gobble you up. Live and catch hold of each moment fully, before it rushes past you.

Less is often more. To freely give what you can to your children, without over-reaching and falling short of your aspirations. You will soon know where you can condense your efforts. To give your child self-esteem and value, without having to bake life-size dinosaur birthday cakes, to prove that you love them. Sometimes, a smile is enough, without needing to provide the paraphernalia of material possessions and activities. It isn't necessary to keep pushing yourself to the limit when a child measures happiness in simple terms – whether you are happy and present with them in spirit or not.

## Filling up the gaps

Identify the ingredients of mothering life that give you true, genuine satisfaction. You want to feel good about being at home each day with your baby, so you're not just digging out your feel-good emotions on special occasions and holidays. Of course you won't necessarily dance for joy through your children's bouts of illnesses or burst cheerfully into spontaneous song as you contemplate your household chores. You will always need to manage the stressful complexities of finance, mortgage, career, childcare and your children's nocturnal waking habits. And try as you might, you may never manifest a massage therapist, cleaner, financial patron or Mary-Poppins-like cheerfulness to alleviate daily causes of tension. Yet you can engage more fully in your role, rather than pushing your alter ego away to a distant stratosphere that you hope may be better than the one you are living in now. If only.

There may be another world where the sun is always shining. It remains to be seen if you can bring it nearer to you. Or else find it inside you. By awakening your spirit, you can pour whole buckets of happiness onto the tedious pressures and frustrations of daily living. See the funny side when things go awry, hug yourself when things go right or wrong for that matter, and enjoy being in perpetual evolution. Don't take yourself for granted, the

ACKNOWLEDGING MOTHERING FRUSTRATION

Think about what your priorities are in life. These might include your home, career, children, partner, other family, friends and colleagues. Now think about what prevents you from giving your best to them. This list could be endless, ranging from the dog's disturbing habit of wandering around at night to major financial anxieties about mortgage repayments or future redundancy. There will always be things you want and need to change. Look at the list and decide what needs your immediate attention, regardless of whether you can 'fix' this. Articulating our troubles enables us to regain a more balanced perspective, in the long and short term.

Write down basic action points to get the show on the road and improve the status quo. It's true that nothing may work. Yet even knowing this is better than worrying. Resolution often comes in strange shapes. Putting other jigsaw pieces into place can create a fuller picture than you ever thought was possible before.

good times or the bad. Your child will learn to value how they are by your own example; keep on trying, even when success is evasive.

## Acting out dramas

The nature of the thoughts we have toward our family, friends and colleagues can indicate the general feelings we carry toward ourselves. It follows that when we notice and cherish kindness in other people, we are more likely to appreciate these same qualities in us. Likewise, if we tend to judge and criticize other people, we're likely to be intolerant and harsh toward ourselves. To be able to honestly assess the emotional balance of our relationships, and accept their shortcomings, enables you to be comfortable in your own shoes. To live freely, without comparing where you stand in contrast to others.

It is worth being frank, even brutally honest, when you're slipping into a false way of being that is harmful to your wellbeing. Even when you're so far entrenched into it, that you can't or won't see further than your own fingertips. You can easily spot the telltale signs: the prickling emotions, unease, self-justification, righteousness and imaginary conversations that keep churning around inside your head. Be alert for occasions when your ego tells you that you're right, and see if you also feel this in your heart. Question your motives behind the character traits you're acting out. Our life drama often seems to negate the person we want to be, defeats our higher purpose and grinds down our enthusiasm to do things differently.

Why brainwash yourself into thinking that your part in this story is the most important one. There are many sides to a story. You're just telling it from one angle, from where you're standing. You may have many valid reasons to complain or praise, also to forgive and be forgiven. But you have forgotten these are just one tale. Your life becomes richer and vibrant when you start to improvise, extending yourself beyond the self-imposed limitations of a set script of lines. Who knows, suddenly you may be creating the possibility of a fresh, happy ending to the story you're telling.

## Playing out mothering archetypes

We slip into habitual roles with our children. Some we love, others we don't really like playing. Especially when they lead us into a full-scale dramatic production in our sitting room. We might like to say, 'That's enough; can I now go back to just being me again.' Unfortunately, the emotional momentum can often be too great, and we have to see things out to the grand finale. Of course, there is another option. To take off our costume, forget our lines, be humble and admit we have chosen the wrong part.

Understand how your subconscious motivation carves out deep emotional grooves beneath the surface. Realigning new thoughts into old patterns. You may put on some of the following acts from time to time. Be honest about recognizing yourself in them.

### Carrying a burden

There is some justification in wearing a martyr complex. Sometimes you've got a reason for adopting a 'poor old me' role when you're sinking under new mothering fatigue. There's truth in it. Your body is in shock from childbirth, sleep deprivation and you're still expected to keep life on track. It's virtually impossible to wake up several times a night, go to work and look after children on an ongoing basis, without short-circuiting. It may be cathartic to create a funeral dirge on your imaginary violin. Yet it is also helpful to know when to change the tune. The intensity of this time is not going to last forever. There are small things you can do to alleviate some of the stress and rise up above the weight of your exhaustion, to make yourself feel better and soothe your nerves.

### Running a military regime

The unpredictability of your baby's waking and feeding habits pushes your personal tolerance levels into chaos. You counteract the threat of anarchy by organizing your baby into a tight schedule to tame their living habits. You may start acting like a bit of a control freak, a slave to discipline. You are so busy following your routine like clockwork that you forget to relax and enjoy your baby, whatever time of the day or night it is. Step down from the treadmill, miss a nap or two, be spontaneous and do what you want with baby when you want, not what you feel you should do at any given time.

### Wearing a shield of self-protection

You gave up your body to your baby during pregnancy. And you're now using the rest of your physical and emotional strength to nurture them through these first intense months. You have reached a stalemate; you have nothing left to give. And you may feel desperate to receive something, anything, back in return: a couple of hours of baby-free time, a few minutes with your eyes shut, one night of unbroken sleep. Sometimes, we all feel that enough is enough. Yet still your child wants more. As your defences collapse, you have no choice but to carry on until the point arrives when your children decide that they don't need anything else, for the time being. And then you can breathe out deeply and know that you are fine.

### Putting on the bandage

You've lost count of the times you've been told that motherhood is one of the most incredible experiences of your life. This goes without saying. Yet it doesn't follow that it's always easy, especially when life with your child isn't evolving to plan. They were meant to sleep through the night at six weeks, not wait until six years later.

All life stories have unexpected twists. If you can follow these without complaining, you may find the path to happily ever after. Cinderella doesn't stamp her feet and throw the grains of rice she is collecting at her stepmother and the ugly sisters – even though she is well within her rights to do so. She finds patience and stoicism to make the best of a bad situation. Even when she doesn't know that things are actually about to massively change for the better. Trust and believe that life happens as it is meant to, without constant interference. You don't need to stick bandages onto difficult times, trying to polish and clean things up. Your mothering story is complete as it is. Although you may not ever live in perfection of fairytale proportions, you can find happiness with a child where you least expect it.

## Following your competitive edge

When you feel inadequate and that you're not worth it, you hide your insecurities, by trying to act bigger and better than you are. You lose your emotional centre of gravity, unable to feel the ground beneath your feet. So you want a badge of honour to commemorate your mothering success at getting your child to sleep through the night at six weeks, eat broccoli and

---

UNDERSTANDING YOUR ROLE

We may give strong dramatic performances to our family audience, to prove the validity of the role we are playing. You can't dismantle human dynamics, to the point where you retreat in solitude to sit in a cave, with only your own thoughts for company. You have an integral part to play in your family's human drama. Yet your child needs to be able recognize you are when you take off the mask you are wearing. To know your authenticity is enough. To meet and find your child when it's just you as you are.

pea purée with a knife and fork, and speak fluently at seven months. Stop! You're so busy swimming ahead that you may not realize you're already out of your depth. You are missing the fun of catching the lifejackets thrown by other mothers, to survive having children together. Sure, you may have it easy now. Yet there may come a time when you're the one who needs support and reassurance, that your child is alright and you're doing fine.

## Following the passage of your breath

At times, we don't want to spend prolonged amounts of time with our young child. Time seems to get ensnared in a constant replay of keeping baby entertained. Doing the same thing again and again, without emotional respite. You can feel startlingly intense symptoms of inertia, low energy, lethargy and boredom. You find it increasingly difficult to summon up any real enthusiasm for another round of singing *Wind the Bobbin Up*, despite your baby's tangible delight in the song and actions. The truth is that at some point, you stopped enjoying it quite as much, even though your baby feels otherwise and would love you to carry on indefinitely.

At this point, we often cast our eyes around for new stimulation, trying to find something else to do. Anything else, except this. Suddenly, we're no longer truly present with our child, but distracted, restless and irritable. We get mindlessly occupied in another unnecessary job or phone call that doesn't really need our attention. We feel mean and useless inside, but we can't stop our attention span and enthusiasm dwindling away into nothing. We readily give into the first sensory impulse that grabs our attention. We don't want to stick it out, or try to focus the mind afresh in engaging with our child. So we create a mental illusion that we need to rush on past this moment, while we actually remain tangled up in our resistance.

## Breathing your way home

You can soften the edges of repetitive emotional strain, by bringing awareness back home to the breath. Give full attention to your breath tone

EXPANDING THE BREATH

The practice of *Pranayama* increases your body's vitality by deepening your conscious control over your breath. Connecting your life energy to the natural rhythm of life on this planet. You may want to seek out the guiding hand of a teacher if you want to understand yogic breathing practices in depth. Yet you can always use the profound power of the breath as a bridge between your mind and body.

through these difficult moments.

Observe the sensation of breath moving within you: the quality of your breath, its length, its depth and the natural pause between inhalation and exhalation. Guide your breath into exhaling smoothly and steadily. Changing the quality of your breath, you give the mind no other choice, but to follow. Sooner or later, your mind comes back to rest in equanimity. Live each breath as if it was both your first and last.

Your practice of mindfulness can drown in the maelstrom of emotions. Yet by following your breath, you can find your way out of the eye of the storm. Through breath awareness, you are led back into higher consciousness. Your mind focuses more easily, and you can sustain longer periods of concentration, without getting tugged elsewhere, while in your children's company.

## Looking at your senses

When the body experiences pleasant sensations, we feel happy, whole and complete. We quickly learn to desire more of the same, seeking out people, objects and surroundings that stimulate these 'good' feelings within us. On the reverse side, you try to push away the things that you don't like. We react strongly to our emotional pendulum at the extremes, actively disliking or enjoying the primary sensation that provokes this. When we are in the neutral zone at the centre of the swing, we gravitate toward what we like best. We want to stimulate something inside us, more intense and

## FINDING FRESH INSIGHT

Sitting comfortably, let your body relax, drawing your mind inward to rest on the breath. Allow your mind to settle and calm, as you bring awareness to the sensation of breath passing in and out of your nostrils. Bring your mind back to your breath flow, the point of your mental focus again and again. It doesn't matter how many times you have to remind yourself to notice the breath. Be patient, calm and observe the touch of breath as it enters and leaves your body through your nose at the tip of the nostrils.

The mind starts to quiet, as your concentration deepens.

You are going to move your mental awareness over the surface of your body, from the crown of your head down to the soles of your feet. Observe any physical sensations: warmth, cold, tingling, tightness, itching or pulsing. It doesn't matter whether you like what you are feeling or not. Keep your attention moving without getting stuck in any one place. If your mind wanders away into distraction, draw your mental focus back again to observe sensations arising and passing. You are not trying to analyze or explain why you feel like this or that. Just witness your true nature.

So starting at the crown of your head, move your attention simultaneously over the front and the back of your skull. Then slowly pass your mind's awareness over your face, around both sides of your neck to the base of your skull, moving across the tops of your shoulders, down your arms and into your hands. Now bring your attention back to the front of your throat, and down over the front of your body until you reach the lower abdomen.

Take your attention to the base of your skull, and start observing the sensations as you move your attention down your back, returning to move it down the central spinal column. Then observe the sides of your waist simultaneously, your hips and buttocks, down both legs, past your ankles, into your feet. Notice sensations arising in the soles of your feet, then the palms of your hands. Finally, scan your body as a whole, and then start

Exercise continues overleaf

again. Continue repeating this cycle of observation keeping your mind as acutely focused as you can. Observe sensations dispassionately, noticing as they arise and change.

Sit for as long as you can sustain relative equanimity. The mind wants to categorize, describe and judge sensations. Notice that your body isn't a permanent fixture, but constantly changing. This person you believe is 'you' is actually in a constant state of flux and transition. You can't hold on to a solid sense of a reality, fixed within the physical mind and body anymore than you can catch the moon's reflection in a pool of water or find the end of a rainbow. The only constant is impermanence, as your thoughts, sensations and feelings ripple and change into new formations.

memorable than a mere sense of indifference.

The mind categorizes and reacts to the world around us; like a puppet on strings, your attention gets pulled here and there. We bombard our senses with stimulation, releasing a torrent of mindless thoughts and emotions. Seeking out desirable experiences that give happy and pleasant feelings, while avoiding and fearing everything else. We rarely get lasting satisfaction. No sooner have you processed one thing, than the mind moves onto something else. Your attention flickers from object to object, searching for something more constant than the changing impressions of the world around you.

*Vipassana* meditation is the practice of self-observation, taught by Gautama Buddha, to help us to see things as they really are. In gaining insight into the nature of mind, you can understand how you relate to a changing world of impermanence. This cultivation of mindfulness is a means to raising consciousness of what is.

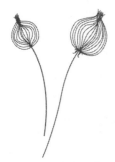

# RELATIONSHIPS AT HOME

*'Even as a mother protects with her life*
*Her child, her only child,*
*So with a boundless heart*
*Should one cherish all living beings;*
*Radiating kindness over the entire world*
*Spreading upward to the skies,*
*And downward to the depths . . .'*
**Gautama Buddha,** *Karaniyametta Sutta*

You may feel like a ship that is barely afloat when you're struggling to cope with the intensity of new motherhood – constantly in danger of capsizing, especially when the rest of the family jumps aboard. You valiantly try to meet your children's needs, (never mind your own), and to balance out the different spheres of your life. You're managing, just about, while your nucleus evolves around your immediate nuclear family. It's when friends and relations arrive on the scene, no names mentioned, that the shifting dynamic rocks your maternal equilibrium.

So the question remains – how do you manage and integrate certain people into your family, who seem to specialize in disturbing your tranquility and peace of mind? Of course, you could contemplate cutting out the prime offenders with a pair of psychic scissors. It may be messy! Especially as it probably involves erasing your partner upon occasion, along with a large proportion of your relatives and mother-in-law. It's important to consider that they also have a vital role to play in your child's life and and so this isn't likely to be a feasible option.

As long as you draw breath and are in contact with other human beings, the simple truth is that you will always have difficult relationships to survive. Your own children may prove no exception to this rule! So, apart from running away to a desert island to argue with coconuts, you can start by taking responsibility for the nature of your human interactions. You can't control other people's spikiness, but you can decide what ingredients you are adding to the pot. It is through the reflection of our relationships that we open or close a window into our heart. Understanding your feelings when you are in contact with other people is a starting point to building a bridge to reach them.

## The journey of interdependence

Watch your child as they go about their day. Witness how they smile and laugh for no other reason than for the sheer fun of it, because life feels good. As an adult, we often define our emotions and the experiences that they generate, in relation to the people or objects around us. We are unable to see that the source of our happiness lies inside us.

So there is always something or someone else that you can make responsible for your feelings. Except yourself, perhaps. As the moods of our children change, it's too easy to link their behaviour to whether we are feeling positive or not. We believe we are happy because they are acting like angels. And we are disappointed when our children's behaviour is less than desirable, and provokes a reverse, negative reaction. We may find ourselves holding conversations along the lines of, 'If you don't stop doing that, I shall be furious', or 'I'm very sad because you did this.'

Stop torturing yourself and them! You cannot depend on anyone else, to fulfil your desire for a good, happy life. You create your own cycle of suffering, likewise of joy and happiness. Your children can't do this for you. While you are making a powerful contribution to shaping your child's life, you are not a part of them, and they are not a part of you. However much you love and adore them.

## Making space for another child

There are two common fallacies about having a second baby: that it is going to be easier the second time around, and you will now know what to do. For many of us, this is simply not true! A new baby shakes up your existence, consuming as much time and energy as the first one ever did. Only you now have even less of these commodities. One thing you do have is direct knowledge of how hard it can be to look after a baby in the early months. Abandon any wishful thinking that second babies equate to half the work. They don't! You are still going to have the same amount of laundry, feeding, lack of sleeping and crying to deal with as before. Even more so. The difference is that your hands are already full with managing your other child, who is also clamouring for your attention.

Think carefully about what will help you to survive and enjoy looking after another baby, even more than you did the first time around. You can't predict your new baby's temperament, or how you are both going to adapt to these early days after birth. So be prepared to change your mothering style to suit this new little person. Let go of comparisons between your children. Enjoy their differences and uniqueness. They are not meant to be the same. So resist sticking labels of 'easy' or 'difficult' onto them. You might forget to take them off again otherwise, and start to believe as gospel truth what the label says. Instead, accept how things are today, and believe they may well be very different tomorrow.

No one ever said that it was easy to have a family comprised of small children. You are facing the reality of caring for two or more dependent human beings. But as the months pass, your life will feel less intense, and things will get easier again. And suddenly your perspective broadens to include other interests, apart from basic domestic survival techniques. Your older children stop stamping on their doll's head or worse; no longer as outraged about their new sibling's intrusion into their cozy world. They haven't permanently damaged the new baby yet; neither have you! And you find you have enough energy again, to watch a whole show on TV, cook a new recipe, manage an adult conversation for more than five minutes, and reconnect with the thread of your old life that you'd put down.

While you can see the shape of mountains looming in the distance, in terms of sibling rivalries and squabbling, you know your family unit is secure. And in rare moments when everyone is happy, it's really rather wonderful in your world.

## Sharing out your love

You may worry whether you will love your new baby as much as you love your first child – or even like them as much. You may feel guilty about displacing an older child with a younger one, especially if they don't seem too keen on the imminent arrival of a new sibling.

So many of these anxieties stem from an unrealistic expectation about your mothering credentials. You worry that you aren't enough. Yet you will always be able to find new reserves of love and attention to share with each of your children, together and as individuals.

There is no boundary to your love; you can give as much devotion as you allow yourself to find inside your heart. There is no limitation, only what you create in your mind. As love rises up, it flows down into your thoughts, feelings and actions, like a fountain of water spilling over and pouring downward. So stewing on negative thoughts blocks up the vital source of your life energy. Your vitality then becomes like stagnant water in an algae-filled pond. It stops love flowing smoothly. So keep using your heart wisely and things will continue moving toward happiness.

There is always enough love. But maybe too much guilt, worry and doubt, that gets in the way. What do you choose to focus on in your relationships with your children? Do you notice when things are carefree, joyful and working well between you? Or do you immediately hone into the more wonky moments, when you have forgotten why you wanted children in the first place? Catch hold of your moods and see the funny, silly side of your domestic antics. This will lead you back to your heart again and again. Soon you realize that love holds your family together, even when you are too tired to notice what day of the week it is.

You have so much affection to share with your children in subtle words and actions. This isn't about grand gestures, but about the simplicity of ordinary everyday moments: the soft brush of your hand against a child's face, a quick kiss thrown on their forehead, taking the time to get down on your knees to smile and make eye contact with them. Find the patience to truly listen and respond to what they are sharing with you.

## Sibling rivalry

Young baby animals like to scrap and play fight each other. It is a vital part of learning how to fend for themselves as they grow up and are alone out in the wild. On the human scale, sibling relationships give your children coping strategies and resilience, to deal with other people without making life into a contest. Most mothers complain at some point about their children's competitiveness with each other: the constant arguments, disputes, attention seeking and lack of cooperation. Yet this is how children learn togetherness. Not by suppressing undesirable traits, but by developing integrity, kindness and understanding.

To live with another sibling is intensive preparation for managing the demands of other relationships, outside the family sphere. By the time your children reach adult independence, they have acted out family power struggles so many times, that they have become more adept at living alongside a planet full of other egos. They can deal with adult selfishness, without crumbling into pieces. Knowing how to cope with other people's excesses and recognize genuine qualities of trust and cooperation.

On some days, your children's bickering may literally drive you mad, especially after you've tried every conflict-resolution strategy known to woman. Grit your teeth and breathe some distance between you and them before you join the fray. Remember it will pass. It's not always like this.

So why do they continue fighting for attention? Your children already know you love them. They also know they have to share this around. And even if push comes to shove, they do love each other deep down. You might well want to shout at them, 'grow up now', as you try to referee another junior sparring match. The irony is that your children are learning the vital arts of negotiation, diplomacy, patience, tolerance and resolution within these sibling relationship dynamics. So do not feel that you must divide your love up into pieces, when you can multiply it into boundless measures instead. Your children might stop tearing each other apart long enough to realize that they already have enough love, care and attention. It's given freely, and they don't have to fight to win this.

## Losing your partner after childbirth

After you give birth, you fall in love with your baby. At the same time your energy is consumed by looking after this tiny human being. And although you said it would never happen, your newborn baby starts monopolizing the best part of you. As you don't have a 25th hour in the day, your partner inevitably loses some of your time, energy and attention. In fact, some days you barely look up to notice them hovering around somewhere in the background. Unfortunately when you do, you may not then like what you see. And so trouble begins.

You are not the first woman who feels they gained a family, but lost a close and loving relationship with a partner after giving birth. You always said you would never neglect your relationship with your partner, in favour of your children. You know the importance of safeguarding your intimacy and closeness as a couple. And would never sacrifice this in the name of motherhood. You truly love watching your partner engage with your baby, and knowing that you are now a family unit.

Yet, it's not the same anymore. Bringing a baby into your mutual lives together creates its own set of difficulties. In truth, it feels like something is going badly wrong between you both. After a few weeks or months of parenting, you're acutely aware that you're no longer the same woman as you were before childbirth. The man you love has vanished, too, and you don't know if you like the new version left in his place. You're even questioning whether you want them to stick around much longer, or at all. And this is before your baby reaches their first birthday!

## Catching up with parenthood

So here you are. Stuck inside the irony of being in maternal love, yet unable to tolerate your partner's presence for longer than five minutes. You are both unable to stop sniping, nagging, criticizing, arguing and destroying each other with hostility. You're not really sharing your parenting adventure together, and you're aware of being very alone within your new family unit.

Stop for a moment and think about how demanding these last few months have been, for both of you. Appreciate the extremities of this intense rollercoaster of change. It's hardly surprising that your relationship is displaying some cracks over the course of all these ups and downs. The danger is whether you now let these rifts widen over time, leaving you and your partner stranded on separate islands.

Don't give yourself a hard time if you can't find constant harmony living together. Or your partner. You are never going to be the same people you once were. And you aren't going to immediately slip into a new, shared normality straight away after giving birth. What you are discovering is how far these ripples of newborn change spread out, through both of your lives. It takes time to adjust and grow into your new lives together, as you reclaim your sleep, hormonal balance, figure and energy levels. Your partner also needs to adapt to parenthood, so lead each other toward a place of tolerance, patience and rationality. The impact of your new baby hits home, leaving behind a memory of the life you once shared with each other. Yet you're already moving on, inhabiting your new life. Together.

## Looking up to see your partner

In your absorption in your lifelong love affair with your child, it's easy to become complacent and careless, and take your partner's presence for granted. Share your parenting delight with them, rather than making this into an exclusive maternal right. Include your partner fully in the good times, letting them bask *with* your child in the spotlight of your love instead of focusing your attention solely on your child. While a relationship can survive some temporary neglect, it's a matter of survival to widen the circle of your affection and let them back in.

The logistics of looking after a newborn baby (especially if breast-feeding on demand) are that you literally have a baby attached to you a lot of the time. And for the rest of it, you're tied up with other children and making sure the house doesn't fall down around you.

Your partner may therefore not feature very high up on your current list of priorities. Ultimately they are an adult, and able to look after themselves. They can wash, dress and feed themselves without your supervision.

(Although sometimes you wonder!) Yet while this is true, they don't have to become invisible. It can take some time for your new mothering rhythm of life to become second nature. So until this happens, they may be waiting a long time for you to resurface again.

## Identifying priorities

If you haven't already done so, it helps to talk about your shared responsibilities, stresses and expectations as new parents. So you have a clearer idea about where you stand in relation to each other, alongside living with a baby. Remember, it's never too late to start building bridges between both of you. Start now. What can you do to enjoy each other's company again, as well as sharing your parenting adventure?

Your primary parenting focus as a couple is to meet your baby's needs in the first year, and enjoy doing this together. So accept that you may want to put major decisions on hold for the time being. Wait and see how you feel about other long-term aspirations, after you acclimatize to having a baby. You already have enough going on, without adding further pressure. There is no need to rush to uproot your finances, work, social life, ambitions or life direction, unless you really want or need to. This is a natural time for reflection, to appreciate what matters to you both. To strengthen the core of your relationship, without getting bogged down in petty concerns. To learn to coexist with a baby, without suffocating your closeness.

Open up clear lines of communication between you, so you can catch hold of these when you need to get through obstacles such as lack of surplus time, money, patience and energy. You are not going to manage this as a couple, just because you happen to live in the same building. While only passing each other like ships sailing through the night. Keep practicing constructive dialogue, so you give yourselves a fighting chance to like each other whenever possible.

Understand what you need to make your relationship strong, healthy and alive, and to be content as an individual and as a couple. You don't always have to agree with the diagnosis of the other, but you can respect this. Seize any moments you can to laugh, enjoy, confide, to be a friend and a lover again (well all in good time!), as well as being parents of a newborn child. So when your children eventually grow up and give you back your time to spend together, you'll be ready to enjoy this new honeymoon.

## Finding each other once more

Assimilating and accepting the changes of parenthood is a lifelong process, which will sometimes be difficult for both of you. You are probably going to be operating in survival mode until your baby acquires more than a casual definition of day and night. So avoid blame and resentment for unavoidable sticking points. Talk quietly without shouting, resolve to make things easier if and when you can, and show an interest in how each of you is finding things. There isn't any need to score points or engage in verbal Ping-Pong, batting accusations back and forth. You're not going to progress if you get stuck in a rally of 'you do or don't do this', 'my life is harder than yours', 'you don't know how easy you've got it', and 'what do you actually do all day?' None of this actually makes anything better or helps to move things along.

Concentrate on how you can support each other in practice; it is the little things that make all the difference and show that you care. Try to make things better rather than worse, and slowly move into a happier place where you can get to know the father of your child again. As well as talking, listen to what you are hearing. Let your feelings clear and settle, accepting and taking responsibility for them, without excusing yourself from the repercussions if you let them loose.

Your partner wears such different shoes from you. So appreciate how it feels to stand in them. You can only do this when you engage in communication with all your heart. If you are interested in your partner's viewpoint on parenthood, you're one step away from being able to integrate your baby into your lives together, as a joint venture. By alleviating some of the individual pressures that get you down, you'll be able to spread and carry the weight of responsibility more easily between you.

As a mother, you are no longer living a soliloquy. Instead, you are transforming a solitary journey into mutual roles of shared parenting. Explore how best to share your domestic and childcare responsibilities so they work well for both of you. And be prepared to discuss and change this arrangement regularly, so you keep your enjoyment of this incredible experience alive. Reaffirm your shared values, interests, concerns and what matters to you both about bringing up a child together.

## So where did the sex go?
Your partner will almost certainly notice if you aren't very interested in having sex. Yet with the advent of sleepless nights, the idea of any other nocturnal activity may be the last thing on your mind. And if you do manage to get a couple of hours free in the day or night, the only thing you really want to do is to sleep, sleep, sleep.

You are no doubt aware, that your body needs to recover from the physical trauma of childbirth. It takes time to heal. In the early days exhaustion and fatigue take their toll on your sexual enthusiasm. You currently have high levels of oxytocin hormones that turn your body into a milking parlour for your hungry baby. You switch on these hormones during breast-feeding, which inhibits your ovulation cycle, lowering your sex drive in turn. Nature is basically telling you not to get pregnant again until your body is ready to.

If you are breast-feeding, you may lose your desire to have sex until you stop. Until then, you'll have to find motivation, time and ample space. Reconnecting with your sensuality, as the prelude to introducing full sexual activity back into your life. The starting point is to consciously nurture your physical body, putting your senses back together again, at your own pace.

Find physical and emotional closeness with your partner, without having to involve sex as the end product. While your baby naturally takes up a large share of your energy, there will still be some left over to give to each other. Here, you can see what you can do to reconnect as a couple. We all know the statistics of one-in-three relationships breaking down. So give yourself a fighting chance to survive this difficult patch of transition and remain intimate. You know your child would much rather have close, happy parents who are in love with each other, more than not. So take up any offers of babysitting, or else beg for them, supporting your relationship as you can.

You need to reconnect with yourself, in order to be with someone else. Have realistic expectations so you move forward happily, without feeling under pressure to make things perfect. The most important thing is to affirm that you love and care deeply. Let sex wait, if necessary, until you are ready.

## Sharing parenting responsibilities

The division of household chores can mutate into an obstacle course, preventing you and your partner from finding living harmony. Look at an average week in your lives, so you can see who is doing what and when. When you both agree on the basic contents of this, assess how you are dividing up your childcare and domestic responsibilities. The basic difference is that one of you may well be out at work most of the day, and unable to contribute much at home during that time. While the other one

---

**TIME OUT**

At last you've got a babysitter booked, and you're ready to spend your first grown-up evening out together for a while. Don't worry if you hit it off with a full-scale argument. Stepping away from baby often opens the pressure valve, releasing the tension building up inside you. So if you explode into a parody of romance, don't give up. Let the air clear, wipe your slate clean of grievances, forgive and move on without holding grudges. And learn for the next time.

You've both been through a lot together, and it may take a few tries to relax, open up and start enjoying each other's company again. Keep this intention alive and you will keep your relationship growing alongside each other and your child.

---

is largely at home in the first instance, engaged in the full-time job of looking after baby.

Time spent at home, looking after a child, is not time spent lounging around on the sofa doing nothing. Women know this, men sometimes don't! To be at work or home is no easier than the other, and most of the time you are both reasonable and accept this. Step back from the heat of any discussion to the contrary, and remember that your partner may feel under attack. Especially if you imply that he is not doing enough, or is inadequate as a parent. Don't be evil and put him down! Yet if he insists in promoting his opinions, that looking after a baby isn't hard work, let him test out his theory in action. Leave your partner and baby to spend a weekend afternoon or two together, without tidying up or preparing things before. And then he can find living proof about how looking after a baby works in practice.

Try to guide conversation away from recrimination and blame, and focus on what you can both do to make your home life a bit easier for one another. You are both probably tired, cranky and worn out, so you can empathize when your partner wants to sit down and put their feet up, rather than pace around the house with a shouting infant to settle.

On the other hand, is your partner allowed to get truly involved in looking after your baby? You may need to back off when they are bonding with baby, and just let them just get on with it, without getting in the way. What's the worst that can happen? It's not necessarily the mother that knows best. And your baby instinctively knows and responds to this.

## Spare time at home

There is a common social misconception that time spent outside of the workplace equates to free time, in which to do exactly what you want. It can no longer be like this. It's true your partner may need some space to make a smooth transition between leaving work and arriving home. It's hard to jump through the front door and be put on baby duty, without being allowed to take your coat off first.

This is tough, but having a baby doesn't allow either of you the luxury of choice right now. A child needs both of you to be present. Especially in the early months when you're still too tired and fraught to cope with much more than you already do. You've also been on duty all day long, and may need some respite. You might aspire to be a domestic goddess and get your baby washed, fed, settled, with a freshly cooked dinner on the table, all by the time your partner arrives home. Yet we all know this is a guiding principle that may not always work in practice. So be clear. Neither one of you is responsible for carrying the entire family's needs on their shoulders, when you are both around at home.

Appreciate what each of you brings. Don't take any goodwill and effort for granted, becoming complacent. You don't need a certificate of achievement each time you do the laundry. But you do need genuine appreciation and acknowledgement from time to time. Think about how you are so much more willing and able to listen to someone who is nice to you. When you are motivated by generosity, support and love, you both find ample reason to treat each other with trust and respect. Ultimately your relationship will be as good as you let it be.

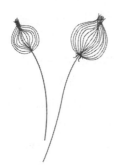

# ANCESTRAL ROOTS

*'. . . We call upon all those who have lived on this earth, our ancestors
and our friends, who dreamed the best for future generations,
and upon whose lives our lives are built, and with thanksgiving we call
upon them to teach us, and show us the way.'*
**Chinook Blessing Litany**

You have given birth to the next generation of your family, preserving an unbroken cycle of life and death that stretches out behind you, into past centuries. Your child now becomes the next link in the ancestral chain passed on to you through your mother, grandmother and their foremothers. If you look at the trail of footprints left by each and every woman in your ancestral history, you can see that all these lives add up to your child's birth in this present moment of time.

This imprint of motherhood gets passed down from mother to daughter, even while each woman creates a distinct life of her own. We are all a product of our times, moulded out of the social and cultural context that we grow up in. Yet we still develop our own unique identity, using the building blocks of conditioning that we create inside us. Daughters carry the maternal touch forward that they receive during the formative years of their own childhood. This legacy of nurture and care has a profound influence in shaping the woman that they grow up into, and the mother they become to their own children.

This skein of maternal love is woven out of women's experiences through the ages. It makes a deep-lasting impact on the emotional development of each successive generation of children. We carry the silent presence of our ancestors within us, even as we make a strong impression on our constantly evolving relationships with our children.

So now, as you stand on the threshold of motherhood, be aware of what you carry with you from your own childhood. And of what is left to explore, maybe resolve, from the emotional inheritance passed down in your family.

## From mother to mother

You can learn a lot about being a mother from your own mother's example, from considering what you liked about your relationship with her while you were growing up, and now as an adult. You may believe that your mother no longer has a direct influence on your life. Yet while you may consciously try to be different, you are still wearing an identity of sorts, made up of the sum of your childhood memories and influences. And your mother was an integral part of this. You may not be able to let go of this legacy, but you can understand it. Your mother was a defining feature in your formative years, for better or worse. As such, parents continue to have a subconscious hold over your adult thought and behaviour patterns, if only as a reaction to be distinct and separate from them.

When you appraise your relationship with your mother, you can understand how difficult it is to always be the mother you aspire to be. Is it fair to shell out blame and judgment, to only notice those things that your mother wasn't able to do for you? Wait and see what your own children think of you later on, when they look back in turn. Appreciate the effort and care that your mother was able to give you, helping you to evolve to where you are now. Your mother is always going to represent and be many different things to you, both now and then. Yet it's most likely that she was only trying to do the very best that she could for you, even if she didn't always score ten out of ten in your books.

KNOW WHERE YOU'RE STANDING

When you look at the current state of your relationship with your mother, explore where things are good, indifferent or downright problematic between you both. The practice of discernment, known as *Viveka*, enables you to look dispassionately at whatever you focus on. Identify the parts of your relationship that fill you with fondness and affection. Where you can see the positive qualities, values and experiences that you would also like to share, enjoy and cultivate between you and your child.

You are already appreciating how you don't always engage with your child without distraction, even though they want this more than anything else. You genuinely want to give your whole attention to your child when you are with them. Yet your mind is often caught up in other things. We remember so clearly those precious times when we get down on our hands and knees and are present with our children. This is as true for you now, as it was for your mother many moons ago.

## So where do you come from?

Your memories of childhood are like a jumbled up collection of sepia photographs with faded edges, which you only notice in passing from time to time. Yet looking closely at past years, you may notice a thread of love running through them, along with other painful impressions, linking then to now. We tend to remember negative past experiences as if from yesterday; they continue to exert a discomforting power and influence over us. Shaking up your emotions into suffering mode, and making you vow never to be taken to that place again.

Siblings and parents have an uncanny ability to cast us back into emotional typecasts that we thought we'd left far behind, long ago. It's all well and good if you have happy, uncomplicated associations with your family. Yet for many of us time spent in our family's company can quickly become unpalatable, disturbing our peace of mind with even a small amount of exposure to them. However, we are unable to swim away from our families, at least not without extreme emotional cost on both sides. You might not choose to see them very often, yet they are still present, if only by their absenteeism.

Most of us hope to mature and shake off the magnetic hold that parents and siblings exerted upon our identity. Yet we may find ourselves falling short of emotional autonomy again and again. Our family has a powerful impact on our lives, reaching beyond the actual contact we have with them. After spending some time with family members, we tend to slip back into behaviour patterns and emotions that we haven't felt since we were ten years old. And try as we might to be grown up and independent, our relationships may seem to remain stubbornly stuck in the same old power struggles, tensions and stewing emotions. Except that you now play these out in more subtle and ambiguous adult guises. It's not great for self-esteem. You think you're doing fine. You are fine; if only 'they' would leave you alone, and let you get on with being fine.

## Resolving your family photo album

So does any of it have to matter to you now? Your experience of family dynamics reminds you to witness carefully the seeds that you're planting and watering now. Translate your insights into practice, as your child grows up and away from you, helping your new family relationships to grow smoothly. Stemming from the centre of love between you, your partner and child. Learn to disentangle and recognize your emotions, especially if they tend to curdle when you're mixing with the rest of your extended family. And remember you're always going to come back to your own home again.

Nobody comes into this earth without a mother and a father. So consciously explore your dynamics with them. Looking at your relations with your family may be one of the most important decisions that you ever choose to make as a parent. You may think that you will avoid passing on the emotional legacy that your own parents gave you. We all hope! Yet you need to know what this is first. It's easy to remain in denial, sidestepping the impact of our childhood at every turn. So pause, step back and acknowledge any past turbulence, and also the love. As your mind slows down to observe your feelings, understand your family's imprint, for better or worse.

The simple truth is that you have spent a large proportion of your life living in daily contact with these people. Although you may never uncover or erase all childhood traces from your psyche, you can become aware of them. You can empathize more readily with how difficult it is to always be a positive role model to your children. So you understand how your family contributes, if only by default, into making you into the person you are now. As you discover the shadows of childhood patterns, you can wipe away any overflow spilling into your new family unit.

Your assessment of your childhood memories reveals what they continue to mean to you. What you love about your past, and what you wish had been different. Step gently into the sphere of your own children's young lives, cultivating a nurturing impact upon their fragile sense of self-esteem. Ultimately your children grow up in the light of your own self-understanding as a mother, assimilating this into the context of their lives.

Reflect on your childhood honestly. You will hopefully find out that your parents helped to plant many positive seeds that grew into a storehouse of self-esteem and wellbeing, as well as many other wonderful qualities. On the flip side, you may discover they also encouraged other traits, insecurities and deficits that you are not so sure about. Which to put it frankly, you feel had an adverse effect on your happiness growing up as a child, creating a sense of ambiguity in your attitudes to parenting now.

Your childhood memories take on a deeper emotional significance and relevance, when your own child's reality mirrors your own recollections. Seeing your child growing up can bring up long-buried memories of your past, giving you clues about how to help them to evolve from this point. It may feel as if a whole new side of you is springing back into life, as you acknowledge the child you still are deep inside, reintegrating them back into your adult form.

## Re-creating childhood through your own eyes

You have the most wonderful gift of empathy to give to your children. You know deeply, intimately, what it is like to be a child growing up. Sure, your personal experience may be like a fossil, buried deeply within your mind. Yet don't forget, you were a child once upon a time. So somewhere inside you, you know the joys and sorrows of being little, young and smaller than the adult world you live in. You can understand how life looks and feels like to your own children.

As a child, you might not have been fully aware, or interested in, the larger historical context unfolding around you. Why things were the way they were. We can only see the impact of society on the microcosm of our family with hindsight. As an adult, you are aware of the driving force of diverse political, economic, social, cultural and global factors shaping the world. You know how a family's fortunes changes the direction of lives,

GOING BACK IN TIME

Think about specific, distinct memories running through your childhood years: your family, the rituals, personalities, vacations, school routines and day-to-day life. What celebrations, occasions and events marked time passing? Remember what it was like, feeling the emotions again within you. Rediscover the different shades and hues, the patterns of childhood events, as you witness your children exploring the world around them now. Let yourself become comfortable with your own past, to connect deeply with it. To know yourself as the child you were once, back then.

Finding kindness and tolerance as you help and support your own children to clamber over similar hurdles of growing up. You can already understand so much of this; you've already been through it before. And while there are many differences, your personal experience can intuitively guide your parenting skills, through your children's lives.

much of which may have passed over your head when you were a child. You cannot change the past, but you can understand what your parents were coming up against. The pressures they faced beyond their immediate control, the larger context of the society you were growing up in.

So this is a reason to revisit the past for a short while. To find out stories to share with your own offspring about when you were a little girl. But you should also recognize and be able to tune into their young wavelength, rather than always expecting them to meet your own.

## Accepting the past

Look at your past with compassion. There is a lot in it that you couldn't do much about. Accept the things that you weren't able to be, that didn't happen, or you would rather have done otherwise. Celebrate the things that led you to where you are now. Understand what you would like to change or do differently. Ultimately, you were only able to do what you actually did at any given time. Not more or less. So accept and forgive yourself when you haven't always done the right thing. Recognize any tendencies to polish up old childhood memories to fit into your desire for a happy ending. There's no shame in having mixed emotions. Whether it's something that happened over 30 years ago, or just a few minutes. It's gone. All that remains is the power it holds over you. In keeping you there still. See if you can perceive a fuller picture of how things were, how they might have felt for other people around you. And if you don't like what you see, well so be it – maybe this is the time to let go and move on.

Ultimately, most of us receive enough love, nurture and goodwill to grow up and thrive, one way or another. After all, we did survive into adulthood, even if we now carry a lot of scar tissue and battle wounds around with us. Your upbringing might have been a bit strange, and not always perfectly delivered. Yet you've also succeeded in bringing a child into the world, wanting to give them your best and to enjoy having them. Surely this is a triumph! You survived your own childhood, and your children will also. So forget the past and its troubles. Instead, concentrate on creating happy, precious memories of family life now for them to pass onto their own children.

## So how did you grow up in your family?

It is probably a good idea to take a look at unresolved relationship issues flying around between you and the rest of your family. You already know when there is emotional tension in the family archives. You feel it at family occasions. You walk into the room, and your emotions wobble away, landing you in a personal version of Dante's inferno. It may be irrational, but you dread the simple act of sharing a cup of tea and a slice of cake with certain relatives like the plague – having to pretend to be civil and friendly when you're seething inside. And this is before they get anywhere near your baby!

It might be worth considering who stirs up your negativity whenever you see them. Look at the imaginary conversations you tend to have after seeing certain members of your family. Where you relish saying all the things that you never would in real life. Pay attention when you fanatically rant on the phone in a 40-minute monologue to friends about the latest family gathering. You know all too well which people make you want to snap, snap, snap with irritation, when you're biting your tongue and holding it tightly inside. You seem to lose all sense of humour, fun and perspective while around them. True, you may not have any issues within your extended family relations. But many of us do. You will know exactly what you really think about them inside.

You obviously can't go to the next family get-together with a big placard that states: 'I have a problem with you!' Targeting the troublemakers with a highlighter pen! But you can resolve this internal schizophrenia of pretence. Admit when you're trying to act differently from how you are feeling inside. It helps to know where you need to mend and patch up the holes in your family relationships, if only to regain your inner poise, grace and balance. When you are living in synergy, without tension and strain, you find happiness. So understand these unhelpful and constrictive family roles, to edge closer to the wholeness you want to find in your life.

## Family hurts

We all tend to hold onto past hurts. It's unhelpful to wallow in autobiographical indulgence, to point the finger of blame, throwing recrimination at anyone else for past offences. What they did or continue to do doesn't matter, unless you let it. Hanging on to it does. Yes, you may have deeply uncomfortable and painful feelings where relationships with parents or siblings definitely broke down. But you will probably also find enjoyable, fulfilling and happy moments past, where you shared satisfaction, joy and laughter with them, that still reverberate in your life.

When you know the nature of your family baggage, you can drop any unnecessary weight that you're simply dragging along for the ride. Wake up and notice where your emotional fault lines lie. We let ourselves be manipulated and dragged down by the subconscious burden of past emotions: jealously, regret, anger and resentment that we insist in carrying along with us. We are so used to feeling as we do, that we don't even realize we are allowing them to become a part of us, and we therefore can't let go.

So don't be tempted to project old secondhand childhood feelings and patterns onto your fresh new relationship as a mother to your child. It's just not worth it. Affirm what you want to do differently as a mother, what you hope your child will pick up from you. If you do bump into old, uncomfortable memories, stay with them for a while. Squirm uncomfortably if you need to, then let go and move on. Leaving the past behind where it is, with as much or little relevance as you want it to have. Apply the insights of what you learn into your present life, to make it worth your while to have gone down the dark alleys of memory lane in the first place. Don't be lazy and repeat old habits. Break the cycle of intolerance, blame and judgment.

Watch how your children behave in relation to you. Do you recognize these patterns in your own emotions? Many of your children's feelings will resonate inside you. If so, accept the residue of your own childhood

---

**REBUILDING A FAMILY CONNECTION**

Has your perception of your mother and father changed significantly since you were a child? What about your relationships with other immediate members of your family? What are the general patterns linking your past and present feelings? Can you find any threads of continuity between your mothering experience and childhood? Would you like anything to be different between you and your parents? If so, who or what would need to change? Do you want to be close to your family? Or are you past caring? What factors contribute to your current feelings?

Clarify how you are weaving the past into current family relationships, and what issues continue to influence your interactions. Identify the childhood you want your child to have: the values, ethics and priorities. Those you will lift from your past experiences, the aspects you want to be different. Look at your family's influence, so you know whether to embrace, change or keep it at an arm's length. Acknowledge the contrasts you create in being different to them.

memories without needing to analyze, dissect and explain them away. So then, you are free to move your mind on to your breath, to being with your child now, not then. Creating a new beginning together.

## Letting go of the past

The space between the past and future brings a possibility of happiness, of awakening into the present. Each day is new, fresh and untouched, if we can be open and receptive to what it brings with it. Yet all too often, we wake up and before we even put a foot out of bed we tarnish its clean surface. Wiping it with the grudges, rages, pride and sadness that we carry from a time before. Tomorrow is still to come. Yet we act like a fortune-teller, predicting the end of our life story before we've read the current chapter.

So what are you dragging after you into tomorrow? What prevents you from catching happiness as it arrives today. We hold onto so much 'stuff' from yesterday, and it slowly gathers strength, accumulating meaning. Is any of it relevant to the person you want to be and know you truly are. You want to make peace with the demons trailing after you. Think about the infinite possibilities of what could then happen. Laugh with, rather than fight them. Untie your mind from its shackles of regret, sorrow, bitterness and see what happens next.

So you are still unhappy, bitter and resentful about something that once happened to you. And you have a choice between singing a mournful tune (which may be very catchy), or trying out something new. Enjoy the possibility of taking a different direction across your emotional landscape. You are now at a crossroads, whereas before you were travelling in circles. Sure, we can always justify the validity of our grievances, continuing to do so until the moon lands on Earth. Sanctifying your emotions in a holy grail of self-justification and righteousness. You may have good reason. But is it worth it? Surely it's a waste of time, destroying the life you have left. You don't have to carry this burden of emotional angst with you into your grave, because you can't bear to be parted from it. Say goodbye. Enough!

We get so used to the repetitive nature of our suffering that we can't let go. We hold on to the negative identity of our pain, like a defensive plate of armour that we wear so often that it melds into our psyche. We mistake the negative vibration of our grievances, hurts, insecurities and suffering for being us. We're so hung up on our past, we forget the art of living.

As each moment arises, it passes. Your mind can move on to that next moment too, if you don't hang on to the one from before. Your baby isn't bothered about why you believe you were treated unfairly back then. There may be grains of truth in what you see, but nothing changes. Protect your truth and integrity. Each time you re-enact your internal dramas, you're feeding the force of negative thoughts and emotions that follow. It doesn't feel good. And you can't then hear much else. Connect with your potential to shine, empowering yourself to be someone else.

When the ghosts of your past take up residence, sit tight. Pull up the roots of negative thoughts and watch your feelings pass. Accept who you once were, the mistakes you made, the grievances received and given, and the things you would change. Then do exactly this. Learn and move on. Staying afloat and present as conflicting emotions wash over you, without getting dragged under in the current. And then, you can sail forward with a new sense of freedom into tomorrow.

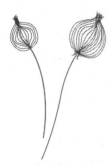

# THE REST OF THE FAMILY

*'May all beings be happy,*
*May all beings find peace and ease*
*May all beings be free from suffering and awakened to the light*
*of their true nature,*
*May all beings be free . . .'*
**Gautama Buddha,** *Karaniyametta Sutta*

There is an old African proverb, that, 'it takes a village to bring up a child.' In many societies, the entire community is actively involved in bringing up the next generation of children. Unlike our contemporary nuclear family unit, where the two birth parents alone carry the responsibility for their child's development and wellbeing. There is a deep-rooted truth in a non-possessive philosophy of parenting. Namely, that a child thrives and benefits from the love, care and attention of many different adults around them, all of whom have a genuine interest and responsibility in their welfare and upbringing.

We may not be able to facilitate a cultural revolution in our society's perspective on parenting, or want to change our attitude toward our extended families. But we can facilitate our children's growing confidence and esteem, by encouraging the constructive input of other family members and supportive adults, other than ourselves. As parents, we were never meant to be the entire universe – the planets, stars and constellations – to our children. They get to know themselves through our immediate nuclear family life. When we allow other relatives and friends into our inner circle, it broadens their breadth of vision, showing where they fit into the world that exists inside and around them.

## Coping with your relative emotions

Do not underestimate the potential difficulties of keeping extended family members happy and content, as well as your baby. To keep communication rolling on a continuous basis, when you are running on an extremely short emotional fuse. The integration of your baby into your immediate family life may already pose a significant challenge. So when you factor in a whole tribe of adults, all waiting for a piece of your baby, you are stirring up a recipe for domestic disaster.

In the first instance, newborn babies are not particularly renowned for their capacity to smooth out the surface of family relations. Everyone loves to turn toward the spotlight on your baby. To admire, coo, cuddle and hold them, and make a lasting impression on their youngest relative. So you've got to be around as mother-in-waiting on these occasions, albeit on an involuntary basis. So there you are, included by default, as relatives settle down and make themselves comfortable. Staking out their emotional territory and personal claim over this tiny grandchild, nephew or niece, or cousin three times removed.

It's not surprising that your baby's arrival exacerbates any reservations you have about involving your extended family in home life. In any shape or form, let alone willingly. Unfortunately you can't live in a vacuum for the next 18 years. So breathe deeply and let the rest of the family in, issues and all. It is your prerogative to then claim your baby and your life back again, when you've had enough.

It doesn't matter if you've clearly got family issues. More important is to stay grounded, so you are focused on making your baby settled and happy. And then you will also feel content and happy. The idea being that this has a positive impact on your partner, other children and the rest of the family, in a sort of trickle-down theory of emotion. This is your immediate priority, and the only thing that really matters over the next few months.

You can't avoid seeing the rest of the family, however much you would secretly delight in this. So the question remains how do you manage tricky relatives? You are already aware that your baby's presence tends to increase initial feelings of aversion or enjoyment toward certain people. No doubt, they also feel the same. Some individuals are a pleasure to be with, others are not. Baby or no baby.

Once you've decided this, unfortunately that individual doesn't really stand a chance against you. It's unlikely you'll ever change your opinion, miracles excepted. It can take years to build trust, a throwaway comment to destroy it. So once your mind is made up that you don't like so and so, this is what you tend to believe, even when it is blatantly unfair to the person in question. You only see this individual according to your personal reaction to them, not in the context of who they actually are. And that's the case even when they would love another chance to play a more positive role in your life.

You inadvertently perpetuate your own angst. You like or dislike certain people with an immediate reaction that kicks in, even before they take off their coat. You see these feelings as originating from this person, not coming from inside you. You push or pull people toward you on the very simple basis of whether you like the feeling-tone of your emotions around them or not. So you're often stuck having to spend time with people you don't like, because they have a prominent role in your extended family. So how do you address the age-old dilemma of what to do with destructive feelings toward a mother- or father in-law, certain siblings or relatives? All of whom have a high stake in your child's development and a natural interest in spending time in your baby's vicinity, and therefore near you.

## Letting in the rest of the family

The doorbell rings, and suddenly you're hosting a whole party of relative issues. And your feelings end up getting bruised and trampled upon. The exclusive bubble of motherhood around you pops, and your mind is left churning with intense feelings of insecurity, hostility, jealousy, frustration and rage at the unwelcome intrusion of other people into your inner sanctum. You may rightly or wrongly feel that your mother-in-law, siblings, aunts and cousins are all constantly judging and interfering in how you are looking after your baby. Implying that they know best, and you really have got it all wrong, dear. And although you don't want to care, you are aching inside from displays of tactlessness and insensitivity projected toward you, the main protagonist in the life of your baby.

Accept when you can't stand other family members who have to play a part in your life. Even when you know you're being irrational, prickly and hostile for no good reason. If you're really in danger of losing the plot, it may help to keep certain visitors at an arm's length from your sitting room until you are sure you can keep a lid on your emotions.

Your child's path is unique. They are going to form strong bonds with relatives, regardless of your personal opinion of these people. Step back from the heat of your emotions, to gain a broader perspective on the dynamics between you, your baby and everyone else. Take yourself in hand firmly when you're overstepping the mark of fairness. Gently disentangle the knot of emotions that you are projecting on to your child's life. It takes a certain grace and courage to admit you can be mean and quite ghastly sometimes. Encourage your children to develop independent and meaningful relationships with other people, whom you may not personally like. You know it's the right and honourable thing to do. Giving your children a foundation of self-confidence and esteem. So they learn to trust their own judgment about others, and grow through the experience of other adults, without needing your constant oversight and supervision.

You don't need to feel insecure, anxious or fearful that someone else is going to displace you from your child's heart. You already know that the more love they are receiving, the more they will grow and shine. Accept the support and help that people have the capacity to give, for the love it is in essence. Try not to judge them for not being you, and what they may miss out in not being so. Notice what they do instead. So much of your aversion stems from your own fears of not being enough. You are giving your child the gift of freedom, to choose whom they like and love, and to be themselves, rather than only exist in your orbit. In doing so, you soften your own vulnerabilities as you accept that relatives are often only doing their best for your child. Just like you.

## Testing communication links

Your baby is a permanent fixture in your life, and involved in most of your interactions with other people. At least until this small third party is old enough to consciously enjoy their own company for a while. So your baby is constantly wedged in-between you and other people. This has quite an impact on your social interactions and conversations, exposing the strengths and weaknesses of your relationships. It feels great when your child reaffirms strong bonds of friendship that you have with some people; where you are comfortable, at ease and able to be yourself, above and beyond being a mother. It's less fun when you feel insecure, criticized and put down, and still have to spend time with these silent enemies.

Your baby is an emotional catalyst, highlighting the strong and weak links in your relationships. You will quickly learn to recognize and appreciate the difference between a friend who lifts your spirits, empowering you to laugh or cry at the funny side of your life with children, and one who doesn't. You don't need social exchanges that make you feel rubbish, where you feel manipulated, attacked or excluded.

## The flood of unsolicited advice

Conversations with family about your gorgeous little baby can quickly revert into a minefield in your living room. However innocuous the subject matter they start from. Casual and insensitive observations about your sweet child's sleeping, feeding or crying patterns can quickly become loaded with subtle critical meaning and inference. You may feel that people are intent on behaving like an unofficial commentator on your maternal performance. You doubt whether they're truly speaking or acting with your best interests at heart. A lot of well-meaning opinion and advice, even if given in good spirit, can easily sound like a negative analysis of your mothering skills. A commentary on what is going wrong, not what you're getting right.

These encounters can make you feel as if you are being squeezed and wrung out like a dishcloth, while you are struggling to remain intact and whole. You always seem to come out on the wrong side of 'happy' family get-togethers. Literally seething with irritation and dislike toward self-appointed experts, who are certain that they alone know how to be a mother, and raise a contented, happy baby.

Alas, as long as your baby is so dependent, you're going to get a lot of different viewpoints on how you should look after them. They are either too hot or cold, wearing too many clothes or not enough, feed too quickly or too little, are crying – so why don't you rush and pick them up? It doesn't matter that your baby's small life is actually rather predictable, revolving largely around eating and sleeping, and doesn't require scrutiny. Likewise, that it's an unspoken rule to never inflict parenting advice onto a mother!

You don't have to take any of this too seriously. You may be given, but don't need to accept unsolicited words. Remember you didn't ask for them! In this way, you avoid increasing your weaponry of anger, resentment or insecurity that you immediately want to fire back at the perpetrator. You can easily manipulate other people's comments to suit your own purposes! Their intention isn't always to harm, even if you're interpreting it like this. They may be telling you, because they care and actually want to help. Don't get hung up on the emotional bait you're given. You are not a fish waiting to be caught! You don't need to rise to negativity. Instead, remain free.

At the end of the day, when everyone else has gone home, you are the mother of your baby. Annoying circumstances will pass until the next time, and then it doesn't have to be so important; dull maybe, malicious no. And the ultimate truth is that you instinctively know what is best for your baby. So it doesn't really matter how you get through the practicalities of your baby's life, as long as you feel and communicate your love to your baby.

## Giving back what you don't need

What does your response to advice-bearers reflect about you? If you are cross, bothered and wound up, let the emotions pass and move your attention elsewhere without taking any of the comments on board (unless there is actually some truth wrapped up in them).

Don't keep any unwanted baggage, but quickly throw it out of the front door after your visitors. Remember, that some people can't help but give advice, regardless of whether you ask for this or not. And there is the small consolation that you may have made someone feel valued, even if you only pretended to listen, and don't accept what they are saying.

You are fully aware that life would be easier if you could get baby to feed, sleep and settle into a manageable rhythm. You are no doubt already trying to do this to some degree, or at least expecting this to happen before your baby reaches adolescence! So you truly don't need to be told this. You might be more than happy to try out of some of the guidance you receive when you have no other ideas to hand about how settle a wide-awake baby in the early hours of the morning. The thing that bossy relatives tend to forget is that young babies, including themselves a long time ago, also woke up several times a night, fussed, cried and wouldn't always go to sleep upon request. Therefore you don't need external scores out of ten on how well you are socializing your baby. You just need unconditional support and acknowledgment that you are doing a great job in your own way and doing the best you can.

## Realizing your true Buddha nature

When you forget your true nature, you cut yourself off from a higher source of life, divinity, love and consciousness. In the context of parenting, you feel a sense of dislocation, unable to see your children's light shining. You are blind to everything. You start to lose touch with your heart's wisdom, acting in the heat of the moment. On occasion, you believe that your child could be a reincarnation of a monster, rather than a three year old testing your boundaries. When you forget to connect to your higher purpose, to find a broader life perspective, you lose meaning in what you are doing. You drift mindlessly through your days, meandering in aimless circles, like a boat without a rudder. It is through aligning our spirit to a higher consciousness, that we fulfil our capacity to live a mothering path with mindfulness.

You honour your beauty, wisdom and humanity when you treat yourself with love, respect, kindness and compassion. You matter as much as anyone else. You cannot wait for someone else to notice this and look after you. It starts right here as you value who you are.

## SELF-PROTECTION

Allow yourself a few moments of calmness to connect to your physical body. Allow your breath to lengthen and slow down, your mind to relax and become quiet. Become present.

Feel your life force expanding, breathing deeply and peacefully. Imagine your breath flowing like light through your body, gathering in a pool of liquid gold at the base of your spine. Breathing in, you create a half circle of light rising up from the base of your spine, over the skull and the crown of your head. Breathing out, you complete the other half of this circle. Light streaming down the crown of your head, over the front of your body, back to the base of your spine. With each cycle of breath, you are breathing a powerful and protective circle of golden light around you. You are safe, held within this beautiful sphere of healing energy; nothing can permeate unless you invite it in. As you breathe energy into this circle of light radiating around you, you become strong and vibrant. You can reflect back any negativity that you don't wish to accept from anyone.

You are surrounding yourself and your child within your breath's sphere. A protective bubble of golden light around you, that keeps you safe and intact from the negative or intrusive interference of the world outside. Trust your intuition that guides you to be the mother you are. Feel nourished, held and nurtured in the warmth of this healing light.

## Self-acceptance

It sounds like a good idea to become calmer, more content and fulfilled. Start by accepting you. Without trying to be a nicer person than you are. Yes, sometimes you are quite mad with rage and irritation, when this or that person acts in a particular way. You do not need to obsess about finding deep and buried reasons, to explain why you are feeling these things. You just are, rightly or wrongly.

So take a few deep breaths, and observe the hue of your emotions. No better, no worse, no more, no less than they really are. Yet always a different picture, from a couple of minutes ago. Notice the subtle variations in the tone of your feelings. Self-analysis can be interesting here, yet it often keeps you tied up in mental knots, without ever loosening the tightness of your emotions. So yes, it's intriguing to notice how unhinged we can be, yet it's stranger still that we're often so busy explaining ourselves, that we never give ourselves permission to actually experience and hold our feelings within us, without trying to rationalize them away. So we repress certain feelings, yet blindly follow these emotional lines into unhappiness.

Your personal route to sanity is to accept the entire spectrum of your feelings, without self-judgment or reaction. That is all there is to it. You can learn to manage your feelings, however wild they are. If you're hopping mad with anger, don't delude yourself that you're not. Black can never be purple. And you'll keep feeling whatever you do, regardless of the stories your mind tells you. So express the content of your emotional journey wisely, until you come to the next slide in this living dream.

Even when you're passionate, magnificent and extreme, you still don't become the permanent manifestation of these shifting emotions. Acknowledge the depth of your feelings with grace, even the yucky ones, without seeing them as a sign of self-defeat or failure. You can't change them. They will dissolve when you embrace them, without pulling away from them. However uncomfortable they make you feel in the heat of the moment. You have courage and strength to face whatever you find within

THIS IS WHO YOU ARE

As long as you draw breath, you will experience different feelings moving through you as things come and go. As clouds move across the sky, your emotions pass through you. You would not try to walk on the surface of a cloud, which appears solid, but is made up of billions and billions of ice particles. You would fall straight through it, back down to earth. Likewise, don't expect or try to make your emotions more tangible and real than they actually are.

Witness the constantly changing landscape of your emotions as they race across the mind's surface. Look closely. You are already feeling something different now from a few minutes or hours ago. You cannot hold onto your emotions, even if you want to; you have to let them go. Otherwise you're clinging onto an idea of something that once was, but isn't anymore.

Self-acceptance is to remain steady when you're up against your strongest, wildest, most depressing sentiments. When internal storm clouds are blowing, and you'd so much rather become somebody else, anybody else, until they pass. To cultivate equanimity is the foundation of resilience. To be able to guide your children to accept and manage their own emotions, without making these into the basis of whom they are.

you, darkness and light, without falling over in horror or despair. Your consciousness becomes something greater and more infinite, than the sum of your individual emotions.

## Finding resolution

In theory, we accept that we all make mistakes, and mess up from time to time. Yet, we often fail to forgive ourselves when we fall short of our personal expectations. Do we even know how to forgive ourselves, let alone those around us? We can easily build a storehouse of past hurts and grievances, without noticing what we're doing. The way to resolution is to become fully conscious of the suffering and pain we're holding onto in our hearts.

It makes sense to practise forgiveness. Otherwise our relationships continue heading off at strange angles, in the direction of recrimination, blame and resentment. We all say and do things that we may regret afterwards. Even if we manage to catch hold of ourselves before we act, we may still need to apologize for our silent thoughts. While we may do so, we still have a sneaking suspicion that we don't really mean it.

We are all well aware that nobody is perfect, ourselves included. Nor is anyone ever going to be. Yet we still take our imperfections to heart, and see other people's weaknesses as a direct affront to us. There are going to be times when we fall way off the benchmark of kindness, thoughtfulness and happiness. Count them and see! It turns out we're very good at exploring our less than perfect sides. Aside from sainthood, forgiveness is a more realistic way of wiping the slate clean. Finding new and creative ways to say sorry to yourself and those around you.

### THE ART OF FORGIVENESS

The world is not out to get you. We're so busy rushing through it that we sometimes forget to see it's basic goodness. It's so easy to only focus on our suffering. You notice your thoughts hardening, and suddenly there is a division between you and everyone else.

Step away from the shadows into light. Create a positive intention. Take mental focus into your heart, as a candle glows brightly, while shadows dance on the walls. It may not come easily. Stand tall and open and feel the warmth of golden light rising inside you.

The same source of divine light is shining inside everyone, even when the shadows are different. You may need to fake forgiveness to start with, to convince your mind to comply with you. It's worth it. To develop your powers of empathy, and know that everyone hurts inside; as well as you. We often want to strike out and blame people for the suffering we feel. Come back to the heart's essence, to the bridge of light shining and connecting you to other people's hearts, and see how those shadows are a part of light.

## Spreading loving kindness

The Buddhist practice of *Metta Bhavana* empowers you to find greater joy and equanimity, giving loving kindness to yourself and all other sentient beings – especially toward people you just can't bring yourself to like. In connecting to your heart, you learn to give love, without exception. Becoming more able to receive love in return, with the same capacity.

The intention is to cultivate a loving, compassionate attitude toward all other living beings without exception. How wonderful it would be to actually feel this, not just aspire to it. Not to confine goodwill to a small minority that you know and actively like. You start by cultivating loving kindness toward individual people whom you cherish and hold close to your heart. Easy enough to do! You then extend this goodwill out to those who exist at the edges, about whom you feel indifference or apathy, or ultimately a dislike or even hatred. Lastly, include the mass of humanity that you don't know, finding goodwill to share with all other human beings, not just a chosen few.

The seeds of your compassion grow and blossom into something larger than the sum of your personal likes and dislikes. You are now connected to all other sentient beings, wishing them well and giving your blessings to them. Your heart fills and overflows, as your capacity to love expands. You are less inclined to feel resentment, jealously and animosity. You can feel you are a part of the universe, along with the rest of humanity. So when you wish for your own happiness, ease and comfort, you wish the same for every other individual, who is actively also struggling to find happiness on the planet. You are no longer alone.

## THE SCENT OF COMPASSION

Sit down comfortably and relax your body, shutting your eyes if you want to. Become aware of your mood, the sensations in your body, and your thought processes. Just accept where you are, without trying to change it.

Draw your awareness into your heart space. Consciously breathe to awaken your heart's energy and feel the presence of love within you. As you exhale, love and compassion flows through your body, filling every cell and particle of your entire being. Take time to breathe. Be peaceful, calm and energized.

Think of someone who you love and care about deeply. It could be someone you know is having a difficult time. Draw an image of this person in your mind's eye and offer them compassion and blessings. Find a sense of goodwill, care and love toward this person, appreciating the qualities you enjoy and cherish in them. As you breathe out, feel a bridge of healing light connect you with them.

Now bring to mind a person who you don't know very well. It might be a neighbour, shopkeeper or tradesman, or else someone you notice passing by. You want to cultivate the same intensity of love and goodwill toward them, giving genuine compassion, as you would to those you already know and like. Exhaling into your heart space, open and connect a bridge over to this person's humanity, letting love flow into their lives.

You're now going to think about someone you don't like at all. Offer loving kindness with the same abundance as you give to those you cherish. Allow your love to flow freely from you to them, without obstacles. You may notice habitual feelings of negativity and dislike trying to grab your attention and get in the way. And it may be that your compassion struggles to remain strong, constant and balanced, against the force of your impartiality, conditioning and limitations.

As you breathe out, keep coming patiently back to the presence of loving compassion that resides in your heart. And gently start again. Feel the warmth of your love and compassion expanding, wishing well to people who really rub you up the wrong way. Feel love as a bridge connecting you to their heart's essence.

Now give loving kindness to all sentient beings: those you know, don't know or don't care about, whether they are alive, dead, dying or yet to be born. As you practise, keep changing who you focus on, known and unknown. Cultivate genuine love, goodwill and compasssion between your small existence and the rest of humanity. You are no longer alone.

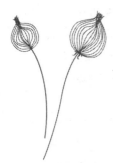

# LETTING IN
# THE OUTSIDE WORLD

'I must extinguish the pain of others, because it is pain such as my own
pain; I must serve others, because they are human beings like me.'
**Bodhicaryāvatāra**

We live in a complex society that gives out contradictory messages about being a mother to our children. On the one hand, you are told that staying at home with your child is the best thing to nurture and stimulate their development in the early years. Yet in the next breath, you're up against the opinion that this doesn't give your child a good role model, as you sacrifice your female identity to the cause of domestic duty.

Stepping away from the simplicity of mutual adoration with your baby, you can feel pushed up against a wall of conflicting values that give a bewildering range of different viewpoints about the best way to go about raising a child.

If society is confused about your parenting role, then what are you meant to think? We can't make head nor tail of the social minefield of bringing up the next generation. We try to discover where our parenting boundaries lie, sifting through an overwhelming and perplexing mountain of childcare guidance and information. And sometimes we forget that when it comes to our children and ourselves, we already know what is best for us both.

You may suspect that your parenting practice is as variable as the days of the week. Your inconsistency baffles you. Something your child quickly learns to exploit to their advantage. Unless you sort out clear values, priorities and ethics that you believe with conviction, you're going to have very lopsided mothering foundations. As a parent, you're providing clear leadership and guidance to your children. Setting constant boundaries in which your small tribe can live and thrive. So they are not left to their own devices, eating ice cream for breakfast, acting as if no means yes and going on strike at bedtime.

You've been waiting a long time for your baby to arrive. Yet despite all the preparation time, it takes several months to truly get to grips with your new maternal outfit, and develop it into a reasonably comfortable practice. There is an assumption that you will bounce straight back into the thick of things after giving birth, and grasp your new responsibilities without any backlash. This doesn't give you any chance to adjust to the miracle of this tiny person lying in your arms. Something you're still coming to terms with. You still have to find out that you can't squash this new baby into an old lifestyle, which comes from a different era. Like a snake shedding a skin, you've outgrown the person you were in a metamorphosis of self-identity. And you're left trying to sew your life back together to create a new patchwork quilt of values – which threaten to unravel with this new soft skein of motherhood running through it.

To remain intact, you have to make massive changes quickly. While giving yourself some slack to adapt to your new maternal status quo. Time to plant out and heel in your newfound maternal responsibility for another human being's wellbeing. You risk tearing yourself into shreds if you carry on regardless, without accepting that you're in emotional transition, in a massive process of becoming something different. You're getting to know yourself again, through the different context of having a baby. Although the world may appear the same, you realize that your place in it is fundamentally different. You've been given a new life to discover, not only that of your baby, but your own.

## Finding your way through the social maze of parenting

As a new parent, you're finding your way through a labyrinth of different social expectations. Learning how to guide your children to grow up, and then live happily ever after. You cannot truly escape from the ubiquitous influence of the media's projection of the contemporary world. Anchoring your cultural conditioning somewhere in the vast spectrum of mainstream society. You may disagree with some of the more controversial assumptions about modern-day parenting practice in the 21st century. Yet you're incredibly fortunate to have the chance to do things in your own way. This is a wonderful thing! Imagine how heavily restricted mothering life was, only a few decades ago. How the vast majority of mothers across the world still have to survive within the confines of autocratic political systems. You're lucky! You have freedom, choice and genuine potential to explore any mothering path you wish to create or take. Use this freedom, rather than conforming to social norms without question.

The social tide of the world will encroach on your family's life, unless you put up clear boundaries to protect your personal relationships with your family. Stepping out of your baby cocoon, your sense of cohesion can shatter into tiny pieces from the force of external pressures and demands made upon you. Believe in your own mothering capacity, and do it your way. There is only this lifetime to make it your own.

Your children have just one mother who will guide them out into the big wide world. They learn to find their way through your reflection within their lives. When you light up their path with your own particular brand of truth and wisdom, you're able to stay on track. You find resilience. Let your intuition guide you, and the world loses its capacity to eat you up and swallow you whole.

When you give out love, you attract it back to you. You cannot feel one thing, then manifest something else, without connecting the two concepts together. You live through your heart space, and become a living example of the qualities you want to pass on to your children. Without lecturing, telling them what to do, or becoming a parody of self-contradiction. If your children can recognize simplicity, courtesy and decency in your shared lives together, they will know how to find and cultivate this, in the world outside. Scatter positive seeds into your children's hearts. So they are living in a mature spiritual garden by the time they're ready to leave home behind them and venture out.

### Regaining your centre of balance

You know that you're a confident, capable woman, able to take on the world single-handed. Well, you used to be like this anyway. Since your baby's arrival, it may be that you hardly manage to get you and baby dressed and breakfasted before ten o'clock each morning. What went wrong with your organization and drive? Motherhood, far from heralding in a triumphant

---

**LETTING YOUR THOUGHTS CHANGE**

Listen to the sounds you hear around you, in the room and outside.
Exhaling, feel your breath dissolve into the air around you.

Release your thoughts, allowing them to vaporize into particles of pure
energy. Breathe out and release anxiety, worries and stress that stake a claim
over your peace of mind.

Let go of old energy and create a new beginning. This is your life now.

---

chapter of female empowerment, has so far meant you barely pass a day
without collapsing into a pile of tears or hysteria. We struggle to get the
simplest of things done, let alone evolving into a symbol of domestic female
emancipation.

Why do we forget so easily to relax and slow down? Instead we get sucked
into the quickening pace of the world rushing past outside the front door.
To follow anything apart from our own mothering intuition is another way
of saying that we are lost. Come back into simplicity. Your children are more
likely to follow you when you live in this place. Like a brood of ducklings
waddling close behind. In a few years, you'll be contending with goodness
knows what: school, friends and other external influences over which you
have little maternal control. So enjoy this time when your children are still
very young, and you are the sun at the centre of their universe. Use this
privilege wisely to help your children grow toward light.

## Material values

Our mothering aspirations can get stuck within the economic grindstone.
We try to keep up with the pursuit of social and material values in
mainstream society; to be an iconic, happy family who have a perfect lifestyle

to match. We all know that money doesn't buy happiness. The depth of our character is the crucial ingredient in raising well-adjusted and confident children. You don't have to give in and succumb to peer pressure. Acquiring a long list of material accessories to reaffirm your child's self-esteem. To assuage your doubt and guilt that you're not giving enough, just being as you are.

Most of us aren't great fans of advertising campaigns that aim to brainwash our child, into thinking they need to have it all. A happy childhood isn't synonymous with smiley-face potatoes waffles, dinosaur-shaped pasta, unlimited electronics, toys that require a wind turbine of electricity, and girls' fashion of pink and purple sequins. Society normalizes a processed and packaged childhood, based on a mission of consumerism. Sending out the dubious message that our child needs to obtain certain desirable status symbols to acquire happiness, and feel completely sated and alive.

---

### CLINGING ONTO YOUR LIFESTYLE

You're offered the chance to spend a week in a castle with turrets and spires, or a run-down apartment building in an urban sprawl. You choose the castle because it looks impressive, without noticing that a witch lives down in the basement. While a fairy godmother has an office in the stairwell of the concrete block, granting wishes to residents.

To be free, stop identifying with your lifestyle and trappings around you. Stand up as you are. Without saying, 'I am this or that sort of person because I have this or that, so therefore I must be so.' You might live in a spectacular house, but does this make you a more beautiful and interesting person? When the carpet is swept away from under your feet, and your possessions go flying, what are you left with? And who are you now? To practise non-possessiveness, or *Aparigraha*, empowers us to let go of any insecurity or delusion; of thinking that we are what we have. Get to know the truth of being you, especially when you have nothing of importance to show. Yet still finding happiness of lasting value in your life.

---

Yet we all want to sustain Earth's resources. To try to leave the planet in a better state than we are doing, if only for the sake of our offspring. We educate our children to make proactive, responsible environmental choices, teaching them about recycling, reusing and reducing non-essential consumption. Yet, we are a bundle of contradictions in practice, compromising our morality when it comes to discerning what we need, possess and want. We boycott grocery-store aisles when Santa Claus appears on the shelves in August. Yet like a goldfish swimming around in circles, we forget our ethical baseline when our children nag us to buy into the latest craze. Even while lecturing our children to eat fresh homemade food, we're pulling into a drive-thru for the fast-food fix, with hardly a moral question mark. One way or another, most of us are going to slip or leap off the moral tightrope of integrating our ethical ideals into practice, at some point.

You don't gain any moral high ground by retreating from the world as it is. You can inadvertently create a lot of tension by living in a vacuum when you have a part to play in a local and global community. Most children want to fit in with their peers and society to some degree. So sure, you can choose to indoctrinate them about the relative merits of healthy lifestyle choices: whole wheat over white toast, fruit over a chocolate bar, water over cordial or fizzy drink. Or expound on the joys of setting up camp in the woods, instead of endless screen time. Yet, you will have the greatest impact on their minds, when you notice, practise and celebrate what is wonderful about human nature in action. When you remove all or most of the props. Knowing also that we may not manage to do this all the time. However hard we try.

## Keeping up with technological progress

A certainty in our children's lifestyle is that technology is embedded into their subconscious minds. A vital, yet possibly addictive part of the world they live in. So to what degree is your child's life governed by it, and can they take it or leave it? Our children display an uncanny knack of navigating their way around this beeping world of electronic devices. You notice how they are using the remote control, while you're still struggling to switch the TV on. This instinctive familiarity gives many children a warped assumption that they have a divine right to unlimited screen time. They are so comfortable in a virtual world of computers, iPads, game consoles, gadgets, tablets and the blasted TV remote, that many feel empty and bereft without it.

It's an undisputable fact that your child's social life could easily evolve around a parallel universe of screen time that fills every spare waking moment. While technological devices have a purpose, they also create a synthesized distance between us and real-life experience on the bare earth. See a beautiful clip of a flock of birds on a Facebook link, or look up into the sky to witness a murmuration of starlings weaving patterns over the land. You become a part of the landscape, or watch it all from a distance.

A lot is at stake here. Sure, your child can find hours of easy entertainment, by simply picking up a keypad. Yet the time spent having a quick adrenalin fix on an electronic device, takes your child away from finding joy, satisfaction and happiness in their surroundings. You may be left in horror at your child's blank, dead stare, after spending two hours on a games console. And can't bear how they seem so empty, restless and discontent without it. So we limit screen time.

After getting instant gratification from the touch of a button, it can be hard for a child to survive in a technological wilderness. They have to work hard, using their imagination and dexterity, to pass over their boredom threshold. To create tangible, fun experiences to keep them entertained and amused. Yet they also regain a natural spontaneity and capacity to interact and create brightness, texture and fun in real-life scenarios. To discover the lasting pleasure of play that is boundless.

You may have to persevere with a child truly addicted to all things that require batteries and charge. Yet you will be able to breathe more easily, knowing your child is engaging all their senses in what they're doing. This is something that lasts far longer than the fading light of an electronic machine, after you switch off the power supply.

So while you support family democracy in principle, you need to enforce certain house rules with dogged persistence and reluctant compliance. As a mother, you are not meant to always do what your children want. Instead stimulate them to live fully in the world around them, rather than taking the easy option.

### The recipe of nature's bounty

We live in a world obsessed with consuming packaged and processed food, with little nutritional value. The more we eat manufactured and ready-made food, the more our children eat a diet with a high percentage of sugar, fats, salt and additives. We create a circle of craving and dependency. This is not to advocate that you ban pizza or ice cream from your freezer. But do not forget to also cultivate a taste for humble, fresh ingredients that might otherwise fail to make it to your table. The nutritional goodness of the earth's bounty can be made more appetizing to your child's palate with a little bit of culinary imagination on your part.

You might already grow your own vegetables, make preserves, cultivate yoghurt, and bake bread and cakes, as a personal lifestyle choice. Yet even so, you don't have to be an eco-warrior fanatic. You're probably never going to convince your child that organic whole foods and vegetarianism is the best way to go when their friends come around to tea. You don't have to handpick caterpillars off your homegrown greens. Or have the time, energy or inclination to do anything more or less, than a weekly food shop for your provisions. The fundamental point is to enjoy the process of preparing and cooking food with love and care, to share with your family. Even, and especially, when dinner arrives overcooked, tasting slightly strange and looking definitely different from the recipe book.

### Family mealtimes

You can enjoy developing your own version of mother earth's kitchen, so it fits into your family lifestyle with grace and ease. You want to enjoy the process of cooking each day, giving yourself enough time to prepare meals without adding indigestible ingredients of stress, anger or resentment into the saucepan you're stirring. So slow down, and feel a connection with nature's produce. Allowing flavours and conversation to merge together at mealtimes. Your body will appreciate this deeply for the rest of your life! And if you find yourself speeding up again, breathe out deeply. Taste what you eat, and enjoy being present with your family, when you're at the table.

An enjoyable ritual at family mealtimes helps to mould your baby's eating habits. If you want your child to eat healthily, and at least like some vegetables, then you are going to have to eat the same as they do, with them. So they can copy how it's done. You might want to take a look at the more decadent eating habits of the adults in your family. Or at least wait until your children are tucked up in bed before you start diving into the cookie jar! You can't munch into snacks of cakes, popcorn and chocolate without your child quickly picking up the message that it's fine for them to do this too.

Let simple, freshly cooked and nutritious food speak to your children, and they will learn to respond with pleasure. Enjoy preparing good meals with love, savouring them with love, and clearing away the debris with love so you're ready to start afresh in a clean space.

## Old friends and new babies

You never thought old friends would be a source of disquiet and upset after you gave birth. Unless you were pregnant in close synchronicity, you may find that you are now worlds apart. In a sense you are. You get pregnant and bang! There go the good old days of sharing a glass of wine or three, staying out late on Friday night, talking for hours any time, and knowing you will drop whatever you're doing to be with them within five minutes.

Once your baby arrives, you can't resurrect this genre of female intimacy in quite the same way. Even after crowning your best girlfriends as honourary aunties and fairy godmothers. Your baby isn't your friend's child, so they're not as emotionally involved with them as you are. The sisterhood may blatantly love the little person, and have a keen interest in your company. Yet they're still one step removed. Unless you all jump into motherhood together, your priorities are going to be different, even conflicting.

Your childless friends are carrying on their autonomous lifestyles as before – without fitting into baby bedtimes, finding babysitters or squashing spare time around a baby's needs. Unlike you! You are a million light years away from those carefree days of adult innocence. Yet, it is more vital than ever to keep the strands of adult friendship alive, now you're a mother.

## Opening the gates of maternal friendship

You can promise that you will never be a self-centred mother, who talks about their child all the time at the expense of being a good friend. Yet your life is running along such a different track from theirs. And your paths may not cross as much as you would like. You are tired, exhausted, with little conversation to give. For God's sake, your daily life is hardly deserving of an explanation. Look no further than the piles of laundry, dirty dishes stacked in the sink and your ongoing argument with the buggy's wheels as they catch your shins in the hall. While friends may mean well, and want to be there for you, they can't always fit into your baby's schedule. Or put you first. So you don't often see them as much as you might like, and are feeling left out. You miss them as much as they miss you! This is big change for everyone.

Your friends with big hearts won't mind if you become a baby bore for a while. They will stop you drowning in the gap between who you were nine months ago, and the mother you are fast becoming. They can talk, listen and laugh you out of any staying-at-home despondency and isolation. For no other reason than they care, love and like you. Even when you misplace your dress sense, go out in shapeless tracksuits, hand them a baby with a leaky nappy (diaper) and fail to apologize when your baby throws up on them. They are happy to put up with all of this, and draw you back into life again. They love you too much to let you go!

When you do meet up, accept you may be back at home way before last orders. You aren't the same person you were in the days before your bump showed. So there is no need to prove you are now.

There is an invisible magnetic force that draws you toward your children. Even when you're having adult respite time and they're nowhere near you. Accept this natural law of mothering, that your children's presence is lodged into your heart. They will always be jumping into your mind, or actually appearing in person to reclaim your attention. More often than not, when you don't want them to.

Your attention is remote-controlled by your children's whereabouts. This is a vital truth of motherhood. Your life is no longer truly your own. Even when they've grown up into teenagers, and are out and about more than you are. You can't fight your children pulling you into their emotional vicinity. There is nothing you can do about this except go with the flow. Accepting that purely adult time is more likely to be the exception rather than the norm, for quite a few more years anyway.

### Catching up with motherhood

Yet life moves on, birthing dust settles and your friends and you learn to retune your social radars to new frequencies. You start to find more snippets of time in which to enjoy each other's company again. Looking back over the past months, you start to value and appreciate the strength of true friendships, weathering and growing. The bonds linking you together develop to fit around your new family priorities. You manage to snatch ten-minute phone conversations and text message chats in your friend's lunch break, while furiously shaking a rattle at your baby to keep them occupied. You're catching up and moving forward in your relationships. And are no longer cast adrift in becoming a new mother.

As you start to get out and about with your baby, you begin to build new relationships with other mothers in the same newborn boat. So don't give up when you feel alone as an adult, but make the effort to find life beyond baby,

> **STRENGTHENING FRIENDSHIPS**
> Enjoy the emotional warmth of being with those you love. Empathize with friends whose lives are complicated. Keep interested. Accept some conversations are going to be interrupted while you orbit around your child's needs. Strengthen the bonds you share with people you care about, as you slowly move through the intensity of this life chapter. Make a commitment to become receptive, open and connected to friends who will nourish and sustain you during your early mothering years.

as well as with baby. There will come a time, when your children really don't live under the same roof as you. And don't want you to be there in quite the same way. You'll then want to enjoy connecting up the living lines of relationships with good friends that you know and love.

## Making a competition out of babies

It would be wonderful if the whole female species became maternal kindred spirits after giving birth. Ready to support and help out other fellow mothers. Unfortunately childbirth doesn't destroy the competitive gene. So baby classes and playgroups are full of alpha females, who believe that their child is vastly superior to everyone else's. These ladies delight in playing a maternal survival-of-the-fittest contest, using poisonous darts of comparison to put others down. Does it matter that your baby is happy lying on their back staring at a dot on the ceiling, while theirs is speaking Mandarin and taking baby ballet lessons. Who cares? You don't have to!

Comparison creates so much doubt and insecurity. Especially in relation to baby development indices, when so much could be at stake. Roses don't worry about coming into blossom in March, at a time when spring bulbs are pushing their stems out of the ground. The leopard doesn't look at the zebra's stripes on the African plains, and think that life would be perfect if they had a coat like that. There is a place for everyone, including alpha females, who may struggle with genuine intimacy. Don't judge others by your own fears of not being good enough. Believe you are doing fine, and your baby is developing at the rate they are meant to be. And most of the time, you will be fine. And baby too. Enjoy life as it comes, living the one you have got, not the one you haven't.

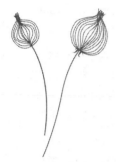

# A WORKING OR
# HOME DECISION

*'Let the beauty we love be what we do. There are hundred of ways
to kneel and kiss the ground.'*
**Rumi**

The thought of your job and career may be the last thing you want to think about, when you pick up your life with a baby in it, after childbirth. You resolutely try to remain in a delightful state of amnesia about the terms and conditions of your maternity leave. Until you arrive at the landmark date you agreed with your employer. Suddenly the prospect of going back to your job or career looms up in front of you. And you really don't know what to do about it. You may be ready to start back at work again, or have no other financial option possible. Yet you might not feel ready, or want to leave home with your baby in it. So you are caught in the balance, trying to decide what is the right thing to do.

You're not at all sure whether you want to be at home, or back at work, and on what basis. Your feelings may change like the wind as you think about this personal dilemma of work or home. Especially when there are significant benefits to be had with both. You may never reach an absolute decision here, coming to a mental stalemate each time you try to think it through. It may be that you only know what you want, after you've dropped off your baby to the child-minder, and are heading on into the workplace. And then you gain partial clarity, on whether you are doing the right thing for you, or not.

## Exploring working motherhood

Many women have conflicting feelings about going back to work. There are so many wide-ranging opinions about the pros and cons of being a working mother in relation to the impact on your child. Only a few decades ago, mothers had little choice but to keep house and look after the children. Whereas nowadays, it's a rarity to be a full-time mother from start to finish. Most of us choose or have to go back to work, at least part-time.

Society currently values a mother's economic contribution to the workforce, more than the unpaid job of staying at home, to nurture the next generation. There is immense social and economic pressure, to be part of a working household, no exceptions allowed. A woman's decision tends to be made from the practical consideration of recouping identity, self-esteem and income. Ignoring maternal instinct. As a result, women are forced to squeeze a demanding career into each 24 hours of the day, alongside being a good mother. And while we try, it's virtually impossible to enjoy both simultaneously, without some sort of personal cost and fallout.

So how do you reconcile mainstream pressure to go back to work, with your emotions telling you it's not such a good thing? The irony is that social research shows us that young children tend to blossom best at home with their mother. Sure, you know you need to work to make ends meet. Yet human babies, along with every other living species on the planet, like to hang out with their mothers in the formative years of life. We intuitively know this, when we drop off our small, vulnerable children at their daycare provision. So we're caught in conflict, between our heart wisdom and the necessity of earning financial security, social status and stability to make life more comfortable. Attempting to find a working balance where everything can fit.

### Keeping a mother's working feet on the ground

Brace yourself to use up a lot of energy and effort to keep your domestic ship afloat, when you go out to work again. This way, you'll be delighted if you can run easily from one end of the seesaw to the other between home and work. Balancing the needs of a small baby with a demanding job can be tricky, to say the least. Especially when managing an oversized proportion of childcare and running the household alongside it. The feminist revolution of the sixties often means little in reality, except women have to work twice as hard to keep a family afloat. There is hardly any quality time together after rushing to and from work, picking up children, doing the laundry, emptying the dishwasher, clearing breakfast things, cooking dinner, clearing up, cleaning, vacuuming, supervising homework, putting children to bed, preparing packed lunches and collapsing into bed; to then wake up and do the same again, six hours later.

Modern lives are complex to manage, bound up in rising variables of inflation and living costs. We never seem able to catch up, keep up or create any slack. Our incomings may never be as much as the outgoings, even when we scrimp and save. We work harder and longer to increase our salary, yet only end up adding more stress and tension to the already fragile relationship between home and the workplace. We seek out a child-minder who doesn't break our heart when we drop our child off to them each morning. Then we burst into tears after calculating what's left over from our wages, once we have paid their monthly bill. Our emotional quality of life declines, as we have less energy, peace and resources to share with our children. We may be able to afford more expensive birthday presents, but we also give less of ourselves.

Yet beyond considering the family's bank balance, many of us still want and need to do something else, apart from staying at home with a child in the early years. You don't want to wave goodbye to your career after childbirth. You may have spent years developing your skills and talents, and really enjoy and are good at what you do. You also need adult conversation, that doesn't revolve around feeding and changing, to stay sane. Are you really meant to sacrifice all this for the sake of your children?

Most of us will decide, or need to have, some sort of job or project to stimulate and keep our adult brain cells alive, over the next 18 years –

**WORKING FEELINGS**

What are your primary feelings about your job and career? Is it a means to a financial end, or something you enjoy and value? Does time pass quickly or drag by slowly? Do you dread going to work, dream about doing something else, or look forward to the next time? What do you find difficult about making the transition into work or home? What would make it easier for you to move smoothly between them both? Listen to what your feelings say each day, about whether you are living in conflict or synergy with your working role. It may take many adjustments to fine tune your working status quo, but you can start moving in the right direction.

while also maintaining a reasonable balance between our working and mothering careers.

## Finding a working balance

There is no right or wrong regarding your decision about starting a job or career again or not. The only imperative is to find a resolution that you are comfortable with, and to change your mind when you need to. You might have thought about your working life totally differently, when your baby was just a concept. So be prepared to adapt and change your plans to suit you now – ideally, organize the situation before you reach your patience threshold. Otherwise you may regret the time spent waiting. You are either happy enough to start working again or you are not. (Except perhaps on Sunday night.) If you can't decide where you are between these two extremes, then explore other feasible options. Cut down your working hours to minimize the time spent away from your children. Consider retraining, becoming self-employed, or creating a job from home. At least for now, think creatively about how to make a living, until you're clearer about what you want to do.

When you assess your lifestyle reasons on an internal scale, weighing up the prospect of going back to work against staying at home, certain individual factors hold more power over you than others. Only you know the true significance of the emotional cost of working against the financial and personal gain, and how much this swings in the balance. To find an individual combination of home and work life, that enables you to enjoy both, without too much conflict. You don't want to feel under constant stress about having to say goodbye to your children. Or conversely dread the long hours spent with them as you realize you'd rather be out at work, compromising the time you do spend in each other's company. Something that is priceless.

Only you know the true depths of your feelings about engaging in a job or career alongside your children. And whether the benefits are worth the loss. Or even necessary. Nothing is ever straightforward. So expect some to-ing and fro-ing until you come to reach a decision that works for you. And remember as your baby grows up, it's likely that it will change again and again.

## Mothering compromises

You might never stop wondering if the grass is greener somewhere else. The sun can always appear to shine brighter on the other side of the street. And good fortune seems to smile in everyone else's life, but your own. To survive motherhood requires the art of compromise. Learning to live with imperfection, so you feel mostly comfortable with your decisions. Without giving yourself a hard time about the parts that you're not feeling so great about. You can always pick holes in your life. So believe in the sincerity of your efforts to do the best you can as a mother for your family. This resolve will get you up each morning, and give you the determination to strive to your utmost capacity, for both you and your children. Knowing that things won't always fit.

You may slip into a satisfying working/mothering relationship, easily carrying your responsibilities at home and elsewhere. You're lucky if you have a saint-like boss who actually helps things along, and tries to make life easier for you. More often than not, mothers face a constant dilemma of juggling their responsibilities. Trying to shave off any non-essential minutes in home and working life, to ensure they coexist without overlapping or pushing the other into disarray. At the end of a busy day, it is you who has to shoulder and reconcile the emotional weight of your dual roles toward your children and job. So this has to be something you can carry without undue stress.

Ultimately you need to get more out of your current situation, than you give up, to make this happen. So keep checking that your current lifestyle choice gives you enough positive outcomes in terms of extra income, stimulating childcare provision, job satisfaction, better quality of free time and adult fulfilment. Be sure that your entire family is gaining enough benefits to counteract the loss of intimacy of a full-time mothering relationship with your child.

You cannot perform this balancing act between work and home without stretching your tolerance and self-endurance levels. And if you come to the edges of your limits, you have to honour and respect them. It is counterproductive to tip the seesaw on a downhill angle, so you're sliding away from equilibrium. Leaving behind all the qualities that help to make life enjoyable in the first place, and worth living.

As you become familiar with the sticking points, you can assess how much you can comfortably carry and cope with, before emotional cracks start showing. You are aware when you are pushing yourself too much, long before you reach meltdown. You can't always force out the edges of your comfort zone, and make yourself stronger than you are able to be. Just because you can't find another way out, or make the impossible happen. Wake up to the truth of your individual capacity to carry life on your shoulders. The fact is that you may not often get into bed before midnight, and rarely run a bubble bath, jumping in and out of the shower instead, just because it takes too much time that you haven't got. Sit down, put your feet up and ask if this is really working. More to the point, is it worth it? Create a decent chance of improving the quality of life today, so you can enjoy

### THE BASELINE OF TOLERANCE

You may be living under a perpetual cloud of guilt and anxiety, worrying constantly about whether you are doing the best for your children. A daily cocktail of stress, you rush around chasing the clock to get to work, get work done, leave work, pick up and drop off children, all to spend a couple of hours with them at the end of the day when you're exhausted and spent. It's a struggle to reconcile two incompatible worlds on difficult days, you may feel you are being torn into separate pieces. Yet despite knowing all this, you still love your job. The dark moments are just a fraction of the whole; you can see and enjoy the bigger life picture, and know it is indeed worth it.

tomorrow when it comes. To work as a means to mothering happiness. This is where you put realistic limits on how much you want and are able to do to guarantee personal fulfilment across your working life.

## Staying at home

You may be delighted with your new domestic lifestyle spent in your baby's company. And decide you want nothing more or less than this. You're not going to be told by anyone that you have to let go of your full-time mothering rights, regardless of financial necessity, or making a bad career decision. You've simply moved on, and can't look back. You want to witness your babies growing up to become little people under your full-time nurture and care. And to learn about yourself in the maternal space you create around you and your children.

Not happy keeping up with the rat race, you're so ready to put it all down, press the stop button and breathe out as life slows down. You skip down from a working treadmill, to make the mothering life you want to experience, before it passes you by. There is something beautiful in learning to simply coexist alongside your children. To be able to pause and reflect on what life is, as you fill your time with looking after your children day upon day, come what may. Each day is a precious gift to learn how to give your best to them, and to receive wonder, joy and delight in return. Getting to know them, through the daily rhythm of spending time with them.

## Mainly full-time motherhood

As time unfolds at your children's pace, you start to explore new potential and possibilities that you had raced past before, without noticing. It's not just having children that changes you; it's looking after them that truly shakes you up. Growing awake through being with your children. This mothering sojourn at home is a personal intensive in getting to know yourself again, this time better than before. The opportunity to stay at home with your children, for at least a few years, is a fantastic, legitimate route, to move far away from the monotony of an unfulfilling career and workload. A sort of personal breathing space to hatch new ideas, and think about what on earth you truly want to do with your resources and talents. To reconnect with a new life when you're not being a mother. And when you're ready to do so again. In the meantime, you've got the most natural and fulfilling job in the world – looking after your children at home, and finding new depths of inner freedom in doing so.

## Overcoming self-doubt

Staying at home isn't the easy option. There isn't an annual leave allowance built into your mothering contract. Some days are so dreadful that you would rather be anywhere, than in the vicinity of screaming fractious children. Most of us have a private catalogue of dreadful mothering moments. When we lose the plot, shout, swear, thump our fists down, sob, stamp our feet, and express just how difficult it feels. We are aching inside, and hate, hate, hate the sheer relentless pressure of giving out to our children. We don't want to! Especially when to put it bluntly, you have nothing left to give. Yet emotions do change again, even if nothing else is much different around you.

Waking up to another day of entertaining your baby, you may succumb to the mothering illness of self-doubt, loathing and regret. Your life with a small baby has probably shrunk to fit into a far smaller geographical circumference. You always need to be able to get home easily since life is governed by feed and nap times. In short, there's far less obvious scope and variety to do what you want in your life, than before. And you wonder what on earth you're actually doing with your days?

You organize a busy program of baby and toddler activities, to try to keep you both occupied from dawn to dusk every day of the week. But even so, you can't summon up the energy to remain steadfastly enthusiastic. You've tried every possible entertainment option available in your baby development guide: a walk to the park, using play dough, arranging a play

WHAT DO YOU ACTUALLY DO ALL DAY?

Don't despair if your partner comes home, and wonders aloud what you actually do with yourself all day. Implying that it's not very much, because they can't see the end results. You're putting your child first, and this is the most valuable thing in the world you can do for them. You're definitely not sitting around having a party. Why is it so difficult for people who don't look after children full-time to understand that it's the opposite of time off work or a personal retreat? You know you're lucky if you manage to eat lunch sitting down, if at all. So value what you're doing. You're shaping the future of the next generation. It's possibly the most important job in the world. And if society acknowledged a mother's true role in securing its wellbeing, the world would be a happier, more peaceful place.

date. Nothing is lifting your spirits. Of course you do manage to plough on regardless. You pass through your boredom threshold to conjure up an enjoyable, satisfying afternoon, making a tent under the kitchen table. However, at other times, you're left craving stimulation or distraction to lift the sheer, excruciating monotony of the clock ticking by, minute after minute.

When you're stranded in this place of lethargy and inertia, unwelcome thoughts rapidly congeal in your head. You start texting working friends, but they're all busy doing important grown-up things, like chasing deadlines, arranging meetings, saving the world and enjoying the hustle and bustle of an active working life. Soon, you're full of self-doubt with gloomy undertones of 'What am I doing with my life?' or 'I am worth nothing,' or 'I could never get a job now,' or 'I have become a nobody.'

## I am worth so much

To constantly rate your mothering experience negatively, means life soon becomes very hard to carry. You question your validity and rapidly descend into melancholy that you are nothing; you're just a mother. Forget the fact there's everything right about this. When you fall victim to desperation, switch off this reel of thoughts, and shake up your energy and motivation. Stop and change the scene.

You are so much more. Start collecting up your low feelings into a pile, to see what they're actually all about. You don't have to indulge your insecurities, inviting them to dine with you. Accepting the downbeat tone of your current emotions isn't going to hurt you, more than you're already doing. Make a friendly acquaintance with your unhappiness, hugging the imperfections that trouble you. Stare at them hard, if you need to. It might make you smile again! Not by stumbling headlong into your negative traits, but by drawing them into the light of awareness. Here they are; that's what they look like.

You can flip over your depressing thoughts like a pancake, to reveal something more positive underneath that will lift your spirits. You may not feel like doing this. It means facing your pain, and doing something about it. Be firm and take control. Just pretend to be a happy sunny person! Your self-doubt runs out of fuel, your positive feelings become genuine, and can move back to centre stage once more.

---

### DANCING WITH SHADOWS

Surround your shadows with grace, humour and beauty, so they have nothing concrete to fight against. Put on music, start dancing, spin around with baby, bounce on the bed, star jump off the sofa, stand outside in the fresh air and fill your lungs. Connect to your vitality, reach up to the sky and get your energy and motivation moving. It takes a firm resolve to change a destructive pattern of self-torture. When your thought patterns shift, you can re-examine your decision to stay at home, and see if you really want to do this, looking at it from a positive place.

Your thoughts are no more alive, than the shadow that falls behind you on a sunny day. You feel so alone with your baby. Yet face-to-face with your suffering, you start cracking open the shell of ego with its walls of pride. Touching the raw vulnerability of the universal condition of living and dying alone. You are the same as the next person beside you. We are all alone.

## Setting yourself free

You don't need to justify yourself to anyone. Why doubt what you already are, by proving that you've compiled an impressive résumé of days spent on the planet. Just believe in and follow the thread of your innate goodness. This is what makes you alive and authentic. As you find courage to accept this, you ignite your heart's purpose with energy, lifting you beyond self-doubt and pain. You spring into life, shaking off the emperor's new clothes of self-importance. Shedding self-identity linked with status, job titles and income bracket, of striving to make a success in the world of externalities. You can stand free, open and exposed, yet courageous and accepting of the joy of just being.

You are something so much more than the string of your accomplishments, trailing out behind you. Your spirit exists beyond anguish, pleasure and indifference. Make your decisions wholeheartedly, and see where they take you. This is what makes you interesting, unique and alive. You can play your emotions skillfully like a violin, creating a song of a life that you want to dance to. All that matters is that you know how to listen to your heart's song, and find your way home.

Once gone, you will never recapture this initial stage of being at home with your child again. So if you do postpone your return to work for a while longer, remember it's just a passing phase of time. It will soon be gone. However, there's equally no point in choosing the domestic option, if you then feel discontented, unhappy and miserable about being at home, day in and out.

Your decision will echo your sense of self-worth and esteem, so you know you're doing the right thing for you. Come rain or shine. And if you are going to stay at home, do it with all your heart and truly engage with your children. Enjoy this wonderful interlude while it lasts. This intense stage of your mothering job is only ever on a temporary contract.

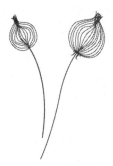

# A MOTHER'S LIFE PURPOSE

'As irrigators guide water to their fields,
as archers aim arrows,
as carpenters carve wood,
the wise shape their lives'.
**Gautama Buddha,** *The Dhammapada*

Inside the spiralling of the mind, there is a centre of stillness and tranquility. Having found this, it inspires you to live with spirit, to know you can go out and find a way to realize your higher consciousness, as a woman and mother. You may never reach the end point. Of filling life up to the brim and letting it overflow. But there will come a realization of inner joy, satisfaction and contentment, in getting to genuinely enjoy what you are doing each day. Regardless of what this is. As you find greater clarity in your intention and purpose, you bring resolution between your highest thoughts, emotions, and their outward manifestation in the world.

The spiritual catalyst, your heart, expands and leads you to cultivate happiness and fulfilment in all you do. Motivating you to find intimacy with friends, invest new vigor in rebuilding a career, to make an effort to fill your afternoon rather than just time wasting. Shattering your sense of adult isolation. Transforming the sheer monotony of spending one day after the next doing pretty much the same thing when you are at home with your baby. Your heart is awakening, and empowers you to be mindful, to see the point of life, when you've missed it.

Your life energy is precious gold dust. Don't waste it waiting for a mythical golden age to arrive, when you are alive today. Is there anything that sets your heart alight when you think about doing it? In your family circle or outside? Coax the dreams out of your thoughts, and take affirmative steps to believe in them. This is what your heart tells you to do, not the arguments why you shouldn't. Your hands may currently be tied down by your baby's dependence. Yet you're building up internal momentum to use your skills, gifts and abilities in this lifetime, not the next one. This will propel you into harvesting the seeds of your intentions, when the opportunity arises. So prepare yourself. Be poised to jump into action when ready. It doesn't matter if it's the sensible thing to do, or the right thing. Tie your dreams to realistic goals, leading you closer toward your life purpose.

Ultimately your life has as much meaning and purpose as you allow it to have. Knowing this, keep finding new reservoirs of energy to fuel your heart's aspirations, to guide you along the path you were born to live.

## Laughing away confusion

There are many reasons not to laugh! You have been pushed through a birthing mangle, and your life turned inside out and upside down. And you thought having a baby was going to be blissful. This must be a cosmic joke! Yet, there is also no reason not to laugh. Sure, you might not chuckle out loud at the intense, graphic nature of difficult mothering moments. But you can find many other things to smile about in delight.

When you look back at some of the low points, see if you can find even a hint of humour in your daily domestic dramas of dealing with small children. Crying babies, raging toddlers and becoming nocturnal may all contribute to curdling your appreciation of seeing the funny side. Yet to be able to find your life amusing, even when you're out of sorts, is the work of a comic genius! Even if this only means a silent smile of irony, as your domestic world implodes around you.

Never forget, you are going to laugh freely again. You will manage to get your life back into a reasonable shape. So grab any chance you can

---

TAKING STEPS FORWARD

Identify tangible goals to help you to achieve your goals and objectives. When you take one small step after another, they add up into a giant leap forward from your starting point. Moving you in the direction you want to go. It's a slow process from birth to acquire the skills, knowledge and experience you need to consolidate raw talent. Whether this leads you to become a quantum physicist, train driver, astronaut or trapeze artist. It's up to you what you make of your pack of cards. You may be crystal clear, or not have the foggiest idea of what your dreams are. Let alone know how to make them become second nature. Find the gaps, and then fill them in. Making your goals into something concrete, practical and achievable. Like climbing up a ladder, rung by rung, until you can see around you, further than before.

---

to soften out the edges, and involuntarily smile at the maverick sides of your maternal escapades. You can either laugh, or else cry. Then hug yourself fiercely for all that you are doing right, and get ready to face the next slide in the kaleidoscope.

## Plant your dreams in real life

Your small children may adamantly want to be a dinosaur or a princess when they grow up. Yet there comes a time when we grow out of a world of make-believe, and look to achieve practical objectives in our lives. We enter into double-digits years, and quickly learn a hard lesson in realism. Try as we may, we're never going to be a prima ballerina, horse-rider or gymnast without application and natural aptitude.

As adults, we grow to understand that we must develop our strengths and gifts to achieve tangible results. You're on a very steep path if you have to invoke flights of fantasy to reach your goals, such as acquiring magical powers or dinosaur wings. So while the sky is your limit, you still need to be able to pluck your dreams from the clouds, and plant them down here on planet Earth.

## Find a definite process to work through

How many days and nights will you give to fulfil your life mission? Without having a loss of faith and interest, or giving up? You can maybe plod on regardless, without seeing any progress for quite a few. But before too long, there are repercussions as your life is batted between your baby and your ambitions. It takes integrity and insight to take meaningful steps toward achieving a personal project. Integrating your goals into your psyche, so they become an instinct. Setting your objectives into a simple, temporal framework. So you can clock your progress, rather than forgetting where you are. If you can measure your success, you're more likely to reach the desired outcome. You can wish on a star, but not much else may happen. Unless of course you manage the star's galactic remit to shine forth.

Set out manageable steps, through clear, structured planning, that you will achieve with reasonable time and effort. Measuring progress clearly after the initial burst of inspiration fades away, and all you have left is hard work, dedication and perseverance. To stay on track even when you're discouraged and don't know whether to go forward or backward.

## Setting goals you can reach

If you're in a hurry to find success too quickly, you may miss a step or two, get lost, and forget to enjoy the process of getting there. Create a clear line of probability, between your goals and reaching them.

As a new mother, you need to create synergy between your personal desires and family harmony. It requires practical creativity to find the childcare, time and reserves to make things happen, outside of safeguarding your children's wellbeing. It doesn't matter if your life efforts aren't worthy of a Nobel Peace Prize. It's worth it, to receive internal satisfaction and enjoyment. Anything less convincing, and you have to question your motivation.

## Changing past records

There is always a possibility to change. You wake up as someone in one mood, and go to sleep in another. Time leaves behind only a trace of what came before. You won't ever fit back into the same mould of nine months ago. This person no longer exists, except in your photograph album. So believe that you can easily change the nature of your life, even with a baby in the forefront of it. The crucial point is to know you are moving on. You can find a life purpose you can enjoy, as well as having a family. The seeds of change are scattered in the instance you look at a new possibility, and determine to visit this place. It's now only a matter of finding a fulfilling way to move in that direction.

If you harness your life energy to your higher wisdom, imagine how much easier life will be, when you believe in what you are doing. To live with enthusiasm, rather than being reluctantly dragged about in the present. You only have one chance at living, so what do you want to do with the day in front of you? It isn't a dress rehearsal for tomorrow. This is the real thing; it's your show, and it is time for it to go on!

You choose whether to be stuck in a rut, repeating the same point in life again and again. You don't need to dance to the same old song; you can change the record. Even if you don't know what it is yet. We no longer believe the earth's surface is flat, and we will fall off its furthest edge. Instead, we know to keep on walking around the earth's circumference as it comes, without ever reaching a final destination.

### Filling up with life's essence

You managed to be born, and to give birth. Now, the only certainty left is death. Yet now you are alive. And until you draw that last breath, you are free to decide how to pass time on earth. Maybe you'll never define your life's purpose. But you can discover what inspires you to feel deep joy, vitality, motivation and interest. To engage in something you truly love doing. Just for the sake of it. So listen carefully to your higher wisdom guiding you toward your life force. This is what you were born to do!

To find clarity of purpose is a choice. We all have times when we are apathetic, floundering among unspoken rules, judgments and fear of failure. We're not good enough or up to the job. We misplace our energy and feel drained and demotivated, moving against the current of our life force. When we understand our resistance, we learn where we need to grow. Ultimately, we only evolve into what we let ourselves become.

When you are on a clear path, life falls more easily into place. You therefore owe it to your children to identify and live out your potential, at least to give it a go. Otherwise our spirit withers away in silent regret, bitterness and resignation that our life was over, before it ever began. There is no need for sadness for all the things you haven't done. Only to rejoice in what you can do now.

> **WAITING FOR DEATH**
>
> A man was traveling on a dusty road when he met an apparition of death dressed in black cloak and hood. He was horrified to hear that death wanted to visit him again in three days time. To take him away from the living world he knew and loved. 'You'll probably need a couple of days to say goodbye,' said the apparition kindly.
>
> The traveler ran to his stable, saddled up his fastest stallion and galloped off as quickly as he could far away into the distance. For three days and nights he traveled without stopping. 'Death will never catch up with me now,' he thought. He only stopped to let his horse drink at a trough as the sun was setting that evening. Suddenly the apparition of death stepped out from behind a bush where he was resting. 'I've been waiting for ages' he said. 'I thought you'd never get here on time.'

## Waking up to the inevitable

It's about you, as much as your child. What haven't you done yet, that you really wish to? What haven't you said that you want to? Do the people you love truly know and feel this? Is there anyone to forgive? No recriminations, only the scent of love. There isn't time to airbrush over the emotional legacy that we leave behind us when we are gone. Affirm what you want this to be in your actions, moment by moment. So it is never too late. Change your parting gifts now, with just a few words of gratitude.

And as for that list of a hundred things you want to do before you die, for goodness sake, get a move on. Start doing some of them while you are fit and able, before you give up temporary possession of this body. Fill your life with fullness. Sharing what is profound, beautiful, silly, funny and poignant in essence with your children. Wake the heart up to the joy and sorrow of being alive. So they can fill their own life with these gifts too.

## Knowing your life purpose

You already know what your life is about. And whether it is all it can be. Somewhere inside, you know. Act on what makes your heart sing, to create a life that you believe in. You start today, sowing seeds of awakening. Listen and become receptive to your feelings, ideas, talents and interests. These insights give you guidance to take your life forward. These are the seeds of your future. When tomorrow does come, you're growing new branches, deepening your roots of resolve.

It may all feel like a million light years from where you are now. And some ideas you may drop and never happen. Yet think of all you could do in the next few decades. Move toward your goals with truth, determination and integrity. Now is your chance to do something, because your heart wants you to. Not because you are meant to, but purely because it feels right to you. You no longer have all the spare time in the world stacked up waiting for you to live. You're caught up in the daily race of keeping up with your offspring. Understand what you want out of life as a priority. And draw your dreams closer to you, rather than pushing them further away.

A clear life purpose is your path to individual happiness and fulfilment. Otherwise you only let your dreams out, during your annual summer vacation each year. When anything seems possible for a fortnight. It's not enough to cram your spirit into a tightly packed suitcase, and then put it away to gather dust in the attic again. You need to be blunt and accept when you've messed up, made mistakes, taken wrong turnings, and want to start again. To resolve the disparity between where your life is, and where you want it to go.

To be a new mother is a fresh chance to focus, concentrate and prioritize what you really believe in, with no more excuses. You mustn't let the miracle of living pass you by like a ship in the mist. Listen to the alarm clock each morning. Wake up from this deep sleep of complacency, and face your mortality. Now start using the life you have left. It is not good enough to live a life of deep compromise, to give up, turn away or do anything else.

In shifting and aligning your life purpose to your heart energy, you create spiritual alchemy to start living out your dreams in the present tense.

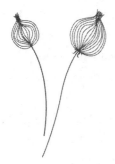

# LIFE BLESSINGS

*'May the road rise up to meet you.*
*May the wind be always at your back.*
*May the sun shine warm upon your face;*
*the rains fall soft upon your fields and until we meet again,*
*may God hold you in the palm of His hand.'*
**Traditional Gaelic blessing**

As you grow into motherhood, you widen your perspective to encompass your children's lives. You meet your baby's gaze of adoration, and step into the presence of love. Connecting you to a higher consciousness, pure, boundless and without conditions. Even when you are so tired and worn out that you barely notice anything else, it refreshes and revives your spirits. And makes life bearable again. When looking after infants, your senses can be lost in a mental fog of physical exhaustion and emotional vulnerability. The mind tries to keep up with the body's needs, often leaving little space to process anything else, apart from tiredness and fatigue. Yet the well of unconditional love still shines within you, waiting to be discovered again.

As a mother, you are blessed with abundance. Your maternal love's breadth is unlimited in essence, unbound by the illusion of separation, division and difference. It links you to the sense of union you felt when carrying your child in your womb. Even though you are both separate individuals now.

## Recognizing the scent of happiness

As a mother, you are given an opportunity to find happiness through the blessing of your children's lives. Each day you experience moments of love and sheer delight, in the minute details of caring for a small child. The way your baby's eyes light up when they see you, how they turn toward your

---

**COMING BACK TO THE SOURCE**

Motherhood possesses an unfailing capacity to lead you back to your heart. Guiding you through the clouds of your emotions, beyond the piles of dirty laundry, vomit and sleepless nights. Your true nature is pure boundless love. We could forget this, yet our children call upon us every day, prompting us to remember it. Calling us to wake up and nourish them with new depths of loving-kindness. Even when the mind resists, and wants to convince you that you have nothing left to give, you can always find more, as the universe replenishes you. To know the source of divinity that runs through everything that you come into contact with. You can never run out or want more, when you quench your thirst with love.

---

voice, nestle their small body into your warmth. Instinctively they look to be with you, in a circle of love. You receive the nectar of bliss. Learning how to surrender and give to this small person, even when every last ounce of strength and resilience is wrung out of you.

Love creates its own healing journey, leading you to the heart. As you find and give love to your children, you will know and drink more deeply from the wellspring of divinity, spirit and benevolence inside. You dissolve your ego-driven obstacles of resistance to meet the challenges of loving your child. There is a natural law of cause and effect: the more love you give, the more you find it within you. You gain a new depth of understanding of how much joy, wonder and nourishment there is in life. Watering your spirit, when the barriers are down. And so the nature of love purifies, evolving under the living force of its own momentum.

Your life blossoms when you grow in love, alongside your children. You may not be doing very much in the eyes of the world, outside your immediate family unit. You might not be able to measure and quantify what you are 'getting done' in your life. At least not using the same terms as before. Yet you are uncovering a new emotional vocabulary, something unique and precious that rings clearly within your heart. You are starting to discover the true nature of who you are, in the clear light of your maternal role, during a lifetime's work caring for your children.

## Coming back home to the heart

Your children's presence within your daily life encourages you to face your ego's reluctance to empathize and interconnect with the rest of humanity. When you collide with your internal doubts and fears, you churn up your thoughts, reflecting dark shadows. Yet we can witness ourselves, without shutting down our heart's energy. We may worry that we're entering into a heart of darkness and may never return. You can understand and transcend your personal sticking points without drowning and giving into your suffering. Even when your nerve endings are screaming out in protest.

This is when you consciously grow, open and expand inside. Taking a deep breath, changing thoughts, raising your vibration, so you still give and receive the best you can. Without doing the opposite. Exploring depths of mindfulness, to come back to the heart as a vessel of love again and again. This is the blessing of motherhood.

You couldn't ask for better conditions for spiritual growth and change, than awakening into motherhood. Even if you took your meditation cushion and yoga mat to a Himalayan mountain retreat for two years in solitude. The catalysts of inner growth are standing at knee height in front of you, as you learn what it means day after day to be a mother to small children.

## Knowing you've got enough

You do not have to ever exist like you're only half-alive. Look at yourself honestly if you're living with eyes cast down, your head and shoulders bent, your spirits low. Are you giving yourself a 'poor old me' storyline? Telling yourself that you will only get a few scraps of happiness, leftover at the bottom of the emotional dregs of your day. All this effort and striving to do the best you can. And yet you're somehow left trying to fill up a bottomless pit of emptiness and dissatisfaction. Your mind can easily believe in the illusion that you are lacking, and there isn't enough to keep you happy on planet earth. The cup of scarcity is never more than half-full, and leaking away fast.

Notice the difference. When the heart is full, it overflows with abundance. When you think it is empty, there is nothing, a void of darkness in which negative emotions take shape. Are you really going to let yourself be disappointed by your incredible experience of motherhood and raising children? Deciding that this too wasn't quite good enough to satisfy your expectations. So you subconsciously create a family life with a greater balance of sorrow and suffering in it than laughter and joy.

Look at the life you already have. Without comparing it to anything else. Sure, fancy cars, clothes, vacations, a large house and wealth may not feature that heavily in it, if at all. Yet, it's already full of so much, overflowing with possibilities of joy and bliss! You've been given a child to raise, the chance to experience the richness of motherhood and the joy of family life. It doesn't matter that you don't have the rest of your wish list when you have enough.

You are fine as you are. Already everything your child wants and needs to be content. Doesn't that tell you something about how perfect you are as a human being? You have all the resources you could ever want to survive, thrive, and also manifest consciousness, joy and peace. To develop creativity, gratitude and happiness by learning to enjoy a larger percentage of each day that you wake up to on this planet. This is the gift of mindfulness, which you can unwrap again and again after birth. To appreciate and be present, awake and engaging in your life experience, creating your heart's wishes, each moment that you draw breath.

### LIVING WITH NEED, NOT WANT

What is on your current shopping list of material happiness? Look objectively at it and decide what gives you a lasting supply of joy and delight? You might get one thing, but suddenly you're not feeling as great as you were, so you want something else. The idea of having an ice cream in the heat of summer appeals much more than eating it in the frost and snow of wintertime, when your enjoyment of it wanes. Yet it is the same cone and scoop; it is us who change.

What would it be like to only possess what is absolutely necessary to survive? The practice of simplicity, known as *Bramacharya*, waters the shoots of fulfilment. You don't have to quench your senses automatically when they're craving gratification. You may want to, but don't have to. This is the vital difference. You don't need to have a life of self-denial, only humble contentment to live with simplicity and sincerity. And to be happy with what you have got. Why acquire more than your fair share, and then some more again. What will it bring? Self-indulgence is spent, and you can't have any more of what you want; it's all gone. And you're left with disappointment and self-loathing, unable to satisfy the dissatisfaction. Enjoy the good times, the feasting, eating and being merry, but don't look to anything outside you to provide lasting contentment.

## Finding abundance

Observe everything that you have of true lasting value in your life: your children, partner, family, friends, work and career, a roof over your head, schooling, medical care and food to put on your table. Decide where to invest your energy and resources to support and enhance your family's wellbeing. Then you won't lose your life's purpose in things that don't really matter that much. When you follow what you believe in with integrity and conviction, you can make a difference in your children's lives.

There is plenty in the world for everyone. You are blessed to live in a democratic society of choices, brimming over with the opportunity to live a good and fulfilling life. No need to be paralyzed by fear that there isn't enough. Cultivate an attitude of generosity, to give back more than you think you can, and see what then comes to you. Share your patience, love and goodwill freely, rather than holding back, just in case.

---

**LIVING IN THE LAND OF PLENTY**

We don't consciously set out to take things from other people. To try to steal a reputation, luck or good fortune that isn't our own. Yet we may want what they have so badly that we leave our goodwill and benevolence at home. We almost wish that things turned out badly for them. Not so much that we then have to feel guilty, but enough so we can regain a sense of superiority and the high ground.

The concept of *Asteya*, or non-stealing, is to give back anything that isn't yours to keep or hold onto. On a literal level, money and possessions that don't belong to you. Also the trappings of success – as interpreted in other people's good fortune, affluence and ease – which you envy and want to have. You compare yourself to another woman and find yourself lacking. You would like to have the beauty and carefree, wealthy lifestyle that you think she has. You want certain things, and resent others who appear to have them. It doesn't seem fair to you. Drop your grasping, and give back good wishes in abundance. Stretching out your blessings all the way to their happiness. Let go of your expectations of entitlement, and be receptive to what you can find to rejoice in that's in front of you.

---

Allow the laws of universal abundance to operate freely in your life. Share what you can willingly without reservations. Opening your heart to love your children, friends and family without harboring worries and reservations that you might be losing out in the process.

You will start to attract internal riches of joy, love, happiness, peace, and fulfilment, far more than ever before. You will then experience life as a boundless gift that you can share, enjoy and treasure with your children and family. No need to measure yourself in terms of social and material standing. The outer shell of your possessions and appearance doesn't really bother you at all. You are overflowing with life's riches. This is the essence of true wealth.

## Being led by mental archetypes

The mind has an entire life of its own. Our mental energy is known as *Prakriti*, and gives movement to our thoughts, emotions and actions. Like a river that never stops flowing, the mind exists in a natural state of constant change, flux and motion.

We express our mental energy through three predominant qualities or *Gunas: Sattva* is characterized by light and purity, *Rajas* by activity and passion, and *Tamas* by ignorance and delusion. The relationship between the three *Gunas* dictates your mind's activity, prompting you to perceive things and act, according to the main characteristic at large. When your state of mind is mainly *Sattvic*, you display qualities of lightness, harmony, peace, contentment and happiness. A *Rajasic* mind is consumed by restlessness, distraction and passion, needing constant sensory stimulation. While when you are in a *Tamasic* state, you show signs of heaviness, lethargy and inertia.

These three primary mental impulses fluctuate and oscillate, in a constantly changing state of balance. It explains why our state of mind changes, when we're still the same person in the same body.

## Correcting myopic vision

Like putting on a pair of spectacles, our state of mind dictates our
interactions and behaviour in each moment, often to the exclusion of
everything else. We don't even notice we live under the umbrella of certain
archetypes, and can only see the world through these lenses. Your mind
is so busy projecting dominant traits outward, regardless of whether
circumstances warrant this. That is until you become more aware, and try to
ensure your mental vibration supports your intentions.

Start reflecting on whether your general state of mind tends to help or
hinder you, in reaching your mothering aspirations. Notice instances when
you are short-sighted, and can't or won't, see beyond your nose. When you
refuse to see instinctive flashes of delight and spontaneity dazzling you with
their brilliance. The mind hypnotizes you to follow certain daydreams, and
you don't even question what you are doing. So your mental activity follows
your emotions blindly, dropping you into negative thought patterns, before
you can notice and scramble out.

Our life unwinds around the same mental qualities that we display inside
ourselves. Circumstances may stay the same. Yet we can strengthen our
natural aptitude for happiness, and notice any mental tendencies that pull us
down to lower frequencies. Drop anything that doesn't help you to cultivate
resolution and harmony. Generate the purity and light of *Sattva* – finding
an energized, relaxed quality of ease – in your mothering experiences. Draw
out your best qualities to share with your children. Understand how mind
functions and become its ally. Using the latent power of positive suggestion,
your ego can become more pliable and receptive. You're able to lead the
mind where you want it to be, rather than getting dragged into negative
places. You are taming the mind's energy and taking the sting out of your
ego's scorpion tail. Your ego starts to listen and cooperate, working with you
to express abundance.

## Raising your frequency

You wake up and wish you didn't have to! You feel run down and concerned that you're hatching a sore throat. You are running on empty, late again, forget the changing bag, get a parking ticket, forget to buy milk. Then baby tips lunch onto the floor and won't settle for an afternoon nap. You're extremely cranky and tired, even more so than baby! The rest of the day passes in a rough blur of fatigue. By the time you cook dinner and put your baby to bed, you're so tired and irritable that you can't see over the top of your negative-tinted spectacles of doom.

Stop and appreciate beauty in front of you. Now! A shaft of sunlight streaming down, your baby's squeals of glee, the expanse of sky above you, the deepening light of evening, the sudden calm of stillness. Countless moments lie scattered through your day, to uplift your spirits and raise your mental vibration to a higher frequency. So stop, notice and find them.

## Appreciating the fabric of life

Take time to feel gratitude for everything you have. Life is tough, extremely tough sometimes, and you may never get that bed of roses to lie down upon. You feel pain and suffering when you're arguing with your partner, are in a headlong battle with a toddler, or struggling to keep up with time. You know this. The stab of anguish and incompletion, when you spot the differences

### FLYING WITH EAGLES

Allow yourself to spread your wings wide open and fly with eagles. When you reach up to the sky, you find that you can see the whole world stretching out beneath you. And then, nothing is impossible!

Create the seeds of your future. You attract the same as you give out. You can learn to manifest your destiny through your thoughts and actions, rather than leaving a trail of empty promises and broken intentions behind you. Today is when you start to create the life you love in the present tense, rather than waiting for another day to come.

between a fantasy world of perfection, and the one you're living on the ground. And so the mood changes.

But the basic truth is your life is still pretty much the same as it was, when you were happy a few moments ago. It's just you've decided to go down a mental cul-de-sac. Even though you know it leads to a dead end. You want your life with your children to be happy and fulfilling. Believe it can be. See that it is. Start focusing on what *is* going right, and leave out all the other 'buts,' and 'if only.'

Appreciate what makes you happy, at ease, calm and whole. You have a wonderful little baby who adores you, maybe a partner who adores you sometimes, and a life that operates above a baseline of starvation. How you perceive the rest of it is up to you.

Why waste time stewing over non-essentials? So what about them! Your sofa is old or the wrong shade, you can't afford a haircut every six weeks, you don't seem to be able to talk to your partner without arguing, and you secretly wonder if life is gently falling to pieces. You could also enjoy what you do have. And build on this. If you examined each one of your grievances, justified or not, you could also find many things to fill you up with gratitude. If only you chose to lift up your eyes and see them. You'd also be able to find someone struggling far more than you are. Look up and notice that life can be pretty ghastly for some people. And they're still cheerful about it. It's easy to fall into a trap of marking life on a negative sliding scale. Yet it's much more fun getting away from this. We take our innate goodness and happiness for granted. In doing so, we destroy the simple pleasures that we already have.

Gratitude starts when you are delighted to be waking up: yes, you did it! You are alive. When you get out of bed, pick up your baby, smile at your partner and find joy. When you greet the day without thinking about what will be wrong in it. When you notice the highest reality of what you can be. When you know where to find more of the good bits and realize that the depressing bits really don't warrant a lifetime of attention.

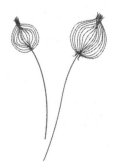

# THE TREE OF
# MOTHERHOOD

*'When the mind is free from the clouds that prevent perception,
all is known, there is nothing to be known.'*
Patanjali, *Yoga Sutras*

As a mother you are growing toward wholeness. It's easy to embrace the good bits. The nice, fluffy sensations of having a child, the maternal equivalent of wearing a soft white bathrobe and wrapping yourself up in warm, cozy feelings. Yet when these pass, what are you left with? The reverse side of the mothering coin, where emotional turbulence makes frequent guest appearances in family life. Unless we change our underlying perspective, we remain stuck too often on this side, powerless to live without tension, conflict and suffering.

To awaken the mind's true nature is to draw life up through our roots, to stretch out branches of our innate goodness and grow toward light. To make a seed grow into a tree, you need to understand the soil you are planting into. Even if it then takes a long time to transform and grow into maturity. Your spirit is opening, expanding and coming home to your family. Weed out the negativity in your inner garden so your spirit can blossom, unbound by obstructions, growing toward joy, contentment and love. And then your children's lives can blossom under the canopy of your protection.

## Understanding the roots of suffering

We'd like to live a happy life. Yet in an average day, there are many occasions when we experience suffering. Where life is less than perfect and complete. It doesn't go according to plan. It might be you, it might be your perception of your children, and it might be your children themselves! It just doesn't seem to add up into a happy family, whatever way you look at it. And you're left feeling misery, pain, insecurity, sorrow, fear, anger, despair, doubt, envy and criticism, even though you don't want this. Only you can change your perspective, to see and do things differently.

To understand the mind is to understand the root causes of suffering. Our mental afflictions, or negative traits, the *Kleshas* prevent us from seeing and living clearly with wisdom. Mental negativity is like grey dense clouds covering a dull, leaden sky. Although we know the sun is burning brightly beyond, we can't see it. Yet we have faith that it is there.

Our true nature of mind is like radiant light. It shines brilliantly even when the surface is overcast with cloudy emotions. If you identity with negativity, you create a prison in your mind, trapping your divinity in a downward spiral of unhappiness. As surely as suffering arises from ignorance and delusion, so happiness arises, when you uncover spaciousness and contentment. You can see through the illusion of reality, letting go of unwholesome emotions, without letting them obscure your inner vision.

To know ourselves: this can only help us to enjoy all aspects of motherhood, without losing our path, or our children, within the quagmire of our mind. To focus on the bliss and joy of conscious mothering can only make the difficult patches easier to carry. The escape route is to understand the nature of human suffering, as this manifests in you. To catch your desire and aversion before the mind is dragged into it. This is the key to unlocking mindfulness.

## Letting go of permanence

All human suffering stems from ignorance, or *Avidya*, that stops us from understanding that life is impermanent, constantly changing. We exist as if our living breath is a possession that we rightfully own. Yet what do we carry with us after death, when this life is no longer in our body? We don't have invincible, immortal powers to keep hold of our children, partners and possessions. At least, not to the absolute degree we might like. We may never find the security we are looking for in life, that things remain the same. Everyday we are getting older, moving toward our death. Our baby is already growing toward this point, no longer as newborn as they were.

So things change, and there's nothing we can do about this. Yet we continue to suffer because we try to keep up an illusion that we're the one who's really in control of our destiny. We're not. We're just a part of the universe. Our children's moods change like lightning, our own moods change, the weather turns, and we're suddenly stuck in a gale with sheeting rain. What can you do, except let go of what was, and accept what is now.

This is the nature of impermanence. We cannot guarantee and predict what happens next, as life keeps moving on around us. We are hot, then cold, happy then sad, often in the space of a few minutes. We process the sensory phenomena constantly changing around us like a jack-in-box. We are this, then that, now we're something else. Our children demonstrate this natural principle of change, letting moods wash over them without leaving a trace. Tears dissolve into smiles and laughter, like the sun coming out from behind clouds, while we are left struggling to keep up with our children's unpredictable natures. We so want things to be permanent and secure, to know where we stand. So we don't let ourselves assimilate change, even when the ground is swept out from under our feet.

## I am that, or am I?

This person we call 'me' is made up of many different personality traits. Creating a shifting illusion of what we are. We project a slideshow of mental images that give definition to the shapes we're forming in our mind's eye. Yet we miss the vital fact that we are not fixed in time and space, but in constant evolution. We're actually not who we think we are, or thought we were.

This illusion of I-am-ness, known as *Asmita*, makes us believe we're a more definite and fixed personality than we actually are. We try very hard to solidify our identity, to be a calm, patient person who never shouts at our children. To persuade ourselves we're really like this, as much as anyone else seems to be. When we really know otherwise.

Family life has a habit of throwing the entire spectrum of human emotion at us. So yes, we may feel contented, as we watch our children playing happily in the garden. Yet in the next breath, we're roaring with rage as this play turns into a sword fight with the runner-bean canes. Afterwards we justify our stream of profanities, saying that it wasn't a true reflection of who we really are. Yet who says you can pick and choose the good bits? You're all of it and sometimes a whole lot more! We will keep on suffering until we stop wearing identity like a cloak, and explore what is constant inside us.

## Unraveling attachment

We know our likes in life, strongly, passionately, and often see this as a sign of strength. The feeling of attachment or desire, known as *Raga*, leads us to need more and more of what we want. So we will experience the 'nice' feeling that goes with having this, again and again. We so like the sensation of certain feelings that we crave them, needing them to fulfil our desires. Without understanding that we are making our happiness dependent on our surroundings. On having everything we want, except learning to be happy inside ourselves. As we can be, when we have nothing.

On a mothering level, it's easy to love the warm feelings of devotion that we get as we wrap our baby up in a soft towel or as their tiny body nestles up against our own; when we are a 'nice' mother. Yet, it's not always like this. We may struggle to reconcile our desire for the good bits, with our resistance to other less salubrious aspects of our personalities. We disown or fight our feelings when we have to battle with the buggy up a flight of stairs, carry car seats with a heavy baby in them, deal with leaky nappies (diapers) in a rush or soothe incessant crying when we want to eat our dinner.

When life doesn't measure up to our expectations, we generate aversion, or *Dvesha*, rejecting what we don't like about the situation. We dislike our unpleasant feelings or sensations, going into battle to try and control or remove them, or else pretend they're not there. Even when our emotions are plainly shouting out, 'Look at us!' Just like the shadows that dominate our nightmares, we struggle to accept those bits of ourselves that we don't respect or admire. Likewise the negative aspects we notice in our children and families. We create schizophrenia inside the mind. A rift between the character traits we like, and those we don't, creating conflict and tension, as we embrace and accept only a fraction of our personality.

## Facing the end

Why do we let these mental traits of like or dislike dominate our lives? At base level, we are in denial of our primordial fear of dying, of *Abhinivesha*.

To accept and live fully, knowing that life is only on loan. Isn't yours to keep. You may nod sagely when you pass a funeral parlour, or Great Aunt Gladys dies at the ripe old age of 94. This is hugely different to integrating the universal truth of death into your everyday knowledge and awareness. To truly accept that death is just on the other side of life. And you are going to die, not necessarily when you plan to. So would you be ready to give it all up, right now, with no regrets? To give each moment your entire attention, knowing it's an opportunity to share courage, certainty and kindness with your children. Adding to, not depleting. They too only get one go at having a childhood, like you did. No trial practice or rerun. Only now.

Once you turn the corner, you can't look back in hindsight and wish you'd done it differently and could you do it again. Yes, there are countless second chances, yet only one moment passing to give love and nurture.

## Planting spiritual foundations

You notice when things are going wrong, and can easily believe that nothing will ever be different. You may feel it is self-indulgent and pointless to look within yourself. So you decide to come back to it later, after baby stops crying. Except you don't. It's sometimes easier to continue as you are, and pretend things are fine really. You live as if you are fast asleep. Yet spiritual growth is worth the effort, and you don't need to be of a yogic disposition. It can't really wait until later. Wake up now! You don't have to be particularly worthy or make any sacrifice to the cause of spiritual transformation. This is about being honest, as a woman and mother. It's about being consciously open and living your hopes and dreams, and realizing what you can be.

We all want to do our best to be a mother to our children. To be a mother that we'd really liked to have ourselves, even if we dearly love our own. Yet we can only be constant in our mothering role, when we get to know ourselves alongside our children. We need to be prepared to change, grow and open to new spiritual possibilities. So we can cope better, even enjoy the difficult, challenging bits of looking after children, as well as the other parts

**SURRENDERING TO THE DIVINE**

We try to be good people, and do the right thing. Yet we may only sense our natural state of goodness in exceptional moments. To touch the divine inside us, otherwise known as *Isvarapanidhana*, is to find the universe inside our hearts. When we're with our children and also away from them. Without measuring our spiritual progress in terms of success or failure. Not looking to achieve a tangible goal of attainment, but trusting where you are. You're not thrown by life's tantrums, including your own. You keep on the path.

As your mothering experience opens to a deeper consciousness, you accept that your life is guided by an infinite source of love, compassion, benevolence and guidance. Something you can't learn, but can only know inside. Your life is unfolding as it is meant to. You're being the mother you are. Surrendering to happiness as it rises up inside you.

What more could you need? Your life is full, complete, overflowing.

we like, and find easy. We need to be able to fill up, so we can give more true, lasting value to our children, family and ourselves. To understand what we don't know about being alive, yet to also find out we're so much more, than we ever thought ourselves to be. Your life begins here.

## Reading a spiritual map

The *Yoga Sutras* of *Patanjali* are ancient texts guiding us inward to make sense of life's dilemmas, and are as relevant today as when they were written 2,000 years ago. Empowering us to develop the tools to find enlightenment, and to cultivate equilibrium, insight and contentment along the way, even if you never reach this ultimate destination. This can only help you to deal with family drama and histrionics over the next 18 years! As your spirit awakens, you gain a new perspective, so you can observe family dysfunction without losing your emotional footing. Knowing the nature of mind, you can steer it back from chaos, anchoring it to consolidate strong family foundations of happiness, cooperation and mutual harmony.

As you put your feet down into family life, you know the path to take. Stepping forward with acceptance, wisdom and gratitude. Opening to each experience you encounter with your children with a staple dose of love, humour, diplomacy and patience. Even if this means that you're reaching again for the cookie jar to restore peace and tranquility in the short-term. To make motherhood into a spiritual practice empowers you to fulfil your true potential to be a wonderful, loving person. To sow seeds of good intention through family life, letting your spirit spread out and flourish, enabling your children to grow up under your mothering canopy of bliss and wisdom. Your heart is singing now, beneath any clouds of stress and tension.

It's worth giving it a sincere go. Rather than not! What other alternative is there, except to make your life yet more difficult because you've run out of ideas? When you put spirituality into your family equation, you start to weave a living thread of happiness and abundance through the individual seams of your family's lives.

## Looking up at the sky from earth

So there are moments of sheer magic in your daily interactions with your children. You are creating beauty and wonder in your interpretation of family life. Who cares that your children aren't perfect, and sometimes seem more intent on deconstructing harmony, than building it. You can still find unexpected moments of clarity and lucidity in domestic chaos by reconnecting to the simple acts of living.

There is joy in transforming the mundane frustrations of motherhood into a living practice of mindfulness. You expand your perspective, as a river widens into an estuary. Your concentration and focus start to burn with the fierce radiance of a star in a clear night sky. You are awakening to your life's purpose, like unpeeling the layers of an onion, unlocking your true potential on this planet.

There is no end-goal to reach. No need to plot your insights on a progress report, to aspire to reaching a plateau of spiritual bliss. All you need is to wipe the slate clean each moment, and live freely with your children with a heart full of creativity and spontaneity. Enjoying innocence, freshness, fun and the adventure of growing together, by getting to know each other again and again.

As a mother, you learn how to orbit gracefully around the parameters of your child's life. You start to enjoy the small details of each day with your children. You learn to breathe freely. To rekindle a child-like spirit of wonder and appreciation, being in your family's presence. To find space around you, like a clear blue sky. To allow your energy to flow smoothly, seen in the microcosm of your domestic sphere. These are the fruits of awakening motherhood; harvested through the daily alchemy of mothering your children with conscious awareness.

## Taking heart from your heart

A happy life starts when you begin to cultivate compassion and kindness. No one wants to be unhappy, yet we manage to achieve this with alarming frequency. As long as we identity ourselves with the body's senses, we set ourselves up to suffer again and again. Capable of great feats of spirit, yet drowning in suffering when the rain starts falling on our picnic, and we don't want it to. There is no avoiding it. At certain points in our lifespan, we all have to come to terms with illness, death, loss and pain. All we can do is enjoy fair weather while it lasts, and accept the downpour that may follow! We may understand that our pathos is rather pointless, yet we keep revisiting it, rather than looking for something different.

Most of us struggle when we see our children suffering. It's hard to accept your children's vulnerability, especially when they're desperately trying to be happy. No one wants to sit back and watch their child making mistakes, messing up, getting hurt or being let down. From relatively minor incidents such as falling down in the playground and scraping a knee, dropping an ice cream, to another toddler grabbing a favourite toy at playgroup. We often point the finger of blame at someone to assuage the pain, often at ourselves.

You're not meant to have all the answers. Or be able to wave a wand that enables your children to know how to stand on their own two feet. You've done a sterling job during pregnancy to protect your baby, giving your own lifeblood to them. Yet after birth, you can no longer have absolute control over your children's environment. You may strive to let your children grow up in a safe and happy paradise. But you will never be able to erase the jagged edges of a world that can be cruel, uncaring and unkind. Sooner or later, they are going to find out that Santa Claus isn't real. Until then and definitely afterwards, you can't guarantee your children's lives will be perfect, safe and sanitized, without locking them up for safekeeping in a treasure chest of innocence.

Our children slowly gravitate away from the living union and wholeness of being in our womb, and inevitably feel a sense of separation. They quickly realize that life won't always provide each and every treat they require upon demand, and they therefore experience some degree of tension and division. You can empathize with your children's suffering as they learn that life isn't always perfect. Yet there's nothing that anyone can do about it. Including you. You can only apply the soothing balm of your unconditional love, reassurance and compassion.

## Applying compassion

As a mother, you experience your children's suffering, as an arrow in your own heart. You try to soften the edges of your children's unhappiness, as if it were your own. The Buddhist concept of compassion, or *Karuna,* is the 'quivering of the heart in response to another's pain.' Yet look closely. Do you really give this same quality of boundless empathy and love to yourself or partner when life is hurting? Feeling your own sorrow keenly without flinching. Until your heart cracks open, you are damming up your own river of compassion.

The Tibetan Buddhist meditation practice of *Tonglen* invites the heart to open and feel compassion toward anyone who is suffering. This may be a

## LIVING FROM THE HEART CENTRE

Sit down comfortably with a few moments to spare. Visualize a person and connect to their suffering, breathing their pain into the centre of your heart. As you breathe in, feel the weight of their misery, anguish and sorrow. Breathing out, allow the healing power of your love and compassion to flow from your heart into their own.

This is the practice of *Tonglen*. While simple, we struggle to remain sensitive and receptive to our other people's emotions. You might experience agitation, restlessness, numbness and anger when you do so. The ego wants to apportion blame and guilt, severing connections with the rest of humanity. Yet in giving genuine compassion without any conditions attached, you find infinite love to share. It no longer matters whether the receiving person deserves it or not. The joy is in giving.

person you know and love, a stranger passing by, or someone unknown to you. The list is infinite.

Opening the floodgates of your own suffering, your heart expands and you allow love to flow through you. You become more aware of the nature of other people's suffering, as well as of your own. You cultivate a deep kinship with the rest of humanity, not only with your children, family and those you love, but also with strangers: the person cold-calling you, the postman, the cashier at the grocery store, the irritating neighbour, estranged relatives, people you haven't noticed yet. In other words, with all of us who are stuck in the same human condition, living its challenges, joys and sorrows together.

Love flows and joy, or *Mudita*, arises in the face of compassion. Breaking down barriers, you feel other people's sorrow as your own. You open up your heart space and feel the joy of love pouring in, as fast as you give it out.

## Cultivating abundance

We enjoy so many of life's blessings. On the other hand, we still excel in suffering, regardless of our good fortune. We all have our individual lessons to learn, which may take us to dark, lonely places. However, the basic denominator is that yes, you are alive. And this is something to be grateful for, every day that we draw breath.

This brings us full circle, to our inter-connectedness with other human beings and the planet we live on. It's easy to wear a comfortable badge of sustainability, deciding to buy organic, fairtrade food, walk or cycle your children to school, and support wildlife charities. We all know enough to appreciate the earth's bounty, and to feel concern when the rains fail and droughts follow in other countries.

Yet go a step further than mere complacency at human desperation. Give blessings to everyone whose lives contribute to your own. Your life depends on the benevolence of humanity, is nurtured by the earth, as much as your baby's small life only exists because of you.

You might recycle cardboard cereal boxes and food packaging with renewed enthusiasm. Stop thinking about the things you can do for a moment. Instead feel a deep-rooted gratitude and appreciation in your heart, for sunshine, rain, soil, the food you eat, the machinery that harvests it, the people who drive the machinery, those who fed these people, provide materials for their housing, and so on. And you're still nowhere close to the factory that makes the cardboard cereal packet that contains your breakfast. It's such a massive thank you to share with the rest of humanity. A life blessing that touches every human being and covers the entire surface of the planet. You cannot separate yourself from a living connection with the universe, as surely as you cannot exist without it. Now think again about how you can lighten your carbon footprint on the earth's surface.

Your life is a microcosm of the galaxy shining above you on a starry night. So coming back home to life with your baby, you can see that your individual life is a reflection of the macrocosm of the entire planet, encompassing individuals, societies and nations living on the other side of the globe. You have a living connection to the universe that embraces the whirring wings of a bumblebee flying out to sea, to see what it can find. There is no part of the universe that you can throw away. You hold the dreams, hopes and aspirations of humanity in your heart, alongside your own. They are all part of the same source of love, however we happen to express this as individuals.

## Making concentration focus

To give your full, undivided attention to your children can be the hardest thing in the whole wide world. Especially when you are distracted by other things, great or small. To be able to turn up our concentration into a single point of undivided focus makes mothering our children a whole lot easier, both for them and us. We don't have to struggle to hold everything in order and shape. Even when our mind is bursting with all the things we're trying to remember and do. Your child gets immense delight and pleasure when you shine your entire attention on them. Without diluting this with the thousand other demands calling you.

Make time to be with your children each day, with nothing else to distract you. Stop diverting energy into answering the phone, texting a response to each and every beep, folding piles of laundry, getting out the vacuum or

---

A CIRCLE OF BLESSINGS

Create a string of blessings, like a garland of flowers, as you go about your day, or through a meditation practice. The simple act of giving out wishes of goodwill and love has no limits. As you bless other people, appreciate how much you have and receive. Extend this stream of light out to touch the hearts of strangers, people you don't like, don't know, or whose lives momentarily touch your own. A sincere intention to wish everybody well; to wish that they too find happiness. When you share happiness, you will notice there is always enough. You can't run out of kindness. In giving love out, you also attract the flow of divinity back into your own heart.

---

chopping onions. Be present without doing anything else, even when there is so much to do. Without making a big internal battle about it.

To give your children your undivided attention shows them they are worth it. Sharing all of your time and energy with them, not just a fraction of it. You don't always need to be getting on with things. Instead, let your child lead some of the time you spend in each other's company. You can simply be there, receptive and open to the presence of this small person, to what they choose to share in this moment with you. It doesn't need to be anything more or less than this.

In this place, your hearts are connected; a bridge of empathy linking you together. The illusion of separation dissolves, and the mind knows the universe inside your child, the object of your perception. This is the yoga of union, or *Samadhi*, where there is no distinction between self and other. You become whole, as your true nature shines out at you.

## Living gratitude

As you wake up each morning, feel gratitude. Allow your life to manifest this affirmation through the day. Let your breath touch your heart and expand your energy outward. What can you give and share? What will make your nuclear world into a happier place to live in? Breathe out and feel your intention merging into the universe. With each breath, reaffirm your

GIVING AND RECEIVING

Moving out to the edges of your generosity, give blessings when you are reluctant to do so. When you are holding back to meet and fulfil your own needs. You can always find something to give. Take small steps to show appreciation to someone: giving a friend a quick call, dropping a friend's children back home even when it's a pain, getting the paints out for your toddler when you don't want to, playing with your baby on your hands and knees, listening to what they are trying to say. You can make a blessing out of anything, creating wellbeing, pleasure and joy and passing it on.

gratitude. Resolving to find inspiration and resolve to manifest this out into your life.

A child's life is a blessing that touches your own life's meaning. When you give birth and become a mother, you receive the gift of nurture and love that comes with looking after another human being. This has the potential to unlock and rekindle your own appreciation, joy, gratitude and zest for living.

To be a mother is a daily wake-up call, a spiritual alarm clock that rings clearly in your life. Reminding you to find hidden potential in every situation that you encounter. You can no longer take life for granted. You are alert and appreciative of the daily miracle of your children's presence; how precious this gift of mothering is. To be alert, receptive and enjoy life with them whatever happens. Come out into the light of awareness and be present. This is all that really matters.

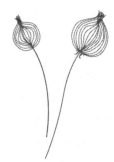

## EPILOGUE

# CYCLES OF CHANGE

*'The butterfly counts not months*
*but moments and has time enough . . .*
*Let your life lightly dance on the edges of time*
*like dew on the tip of a leaf.'*
**Rabindranath Tagore**

You have been given the gift of motherhood, your life intertwined with that of your child's in this lifetime. Not only a life-changing event, but also giving you a profound choice: to use this experience as a catalyst of spiritual awakening and growth. Your child's life is a blessing, and as a mother, you are given an opportunity of connecting to a higher consciousness, looking after them each day. Getting to know the universal spirit of love and divinity in your child's presence. This is your inspiration and muse.

To consciously look after a baby and child requires you to cultivate self-awareness, compassion, insight and focus. This is your starting point and end point. To create an authentic practice of mindfulness out of ordinary family life, that becomes the spiritual essence of your life. It takes genuine integrity, effort, honesty and patience to grow and change. Your child may be one of the most profound and challenging teachers you ever meet. As your heart learns to open with boundless love and compassion, you can enjoy the joys and sorrows of motherhood with greater peace, happiness and fulfilment.

As you slowly move on from the early days of mothering life, you can look back and see how far you have already come. Accepting of the truth you are living right now. Planting fresh seeds of awakening. Expanding your perspective to embrace new depths of joy, wisdom and insight through the daily challenges of looking after children. Just sit down and make eye contact with the small spiritual guide looking up at you.

Follow your mothering path into new cycles of change as the seasons pass. With each day, learn to connect to your present experience, in an infinite process of self-discovery and renewal. Letting go of yesterday. Trusting that everything is unfolding today as it is meant to. Now.

Your life is starting afresh, each day a new beginning. Embrace your true infinite nature, present, alive. As a woman and mother, you can cultivate a living backdrop of love, consciousness and divinity against which you and your family can live and grow. Awakening your spirit through mindfulness.

# BIBLIOGRAPHY

Conze, E., (editor) *Buddhist Wisdom: The 'Diamond' and 'Heart' Sutra*,
Vintage Books, 2001

Desikachar, T.K.V., *The Heart of Yoga: Developing a Personal Practice*,
Inner Traditions International, 1995

Easwaran, E., (introduction and translation) *The Dhammapada*,
Nilgiri Press, 2007

Hawley, J., *The Bhagavad Gita: A Walkthrough for Westerners*,
New World Library, 2001

Nhat Hanh, T., *The Miracle of Mindfulness: The Classic Guide to
Meditation by the World's Most Revered Master*, Rider, Ebury Press, 2008

Nhat Hanh, T., *Transformation and Healing: Sutra on the Four Establishments
of Mindfulness*, Rider, Ebury Press, 1993

Roach, G.M., *The Tibetan Book of Yoga: Ancient Buddhist Teachings on
the Philosophy and Practice of Yoga*, Doubleday, Random House, 2004

Tolle, E., *The Power of Now: A Guide to Spiritual Enlightenment*,
Hodder & Stoughton, 2001

# FURTHER READING

Aldort, N., *Raising our Children, Raising Ourselves*, Publishers Network, 2006

Balaskas, J., *New Active Birth: A Concise Guide to Natural Childbirth*, Thorsons Press, 1990

Freedman, F.B., *Yoga for Pregnancy, Birth and Beyond*, Dorling Kindersley, 2004

England, P. and Horowitz, R., *Birthing from Within: An Extra-ordinary Guide to Childbirth Preparation*, Partera Press, 1998

Thuli-Dinsmore, U., *A Mother's Breath: A Definitive Guide to Yoga Breathing, Sound and Awareness Practices During Pregnancy, Birth, Post-Natal Recovery and Mothering*, Sitaram & Sons Partnerships, 2006